# Don't Wait To Lose Weight

## 10 Steps to Kick-Start Your Fitness Journey

When you need to believe,
start with yourself.

# Don't Wait To Lose Weight
# 10 Steps to Kick-Start
# Your Fitness Journey

Saideh Browne

GS Publishing Group
New York City, New York

## Saideh's Books

Win From Within

Embrace The Heat

Fit Girl Fabulous

Don't Wait To Lose Weight!

SheEO's Rock! 99 Tips
To Transform Your Business Today

From Hip-Hop to Heaven for Girls

From Hip-Hop to Heaven

Can Hip-Hop be Holy?

100 Words of Wisdom for Women

Life Remixed: Understanding
the Journey of Success

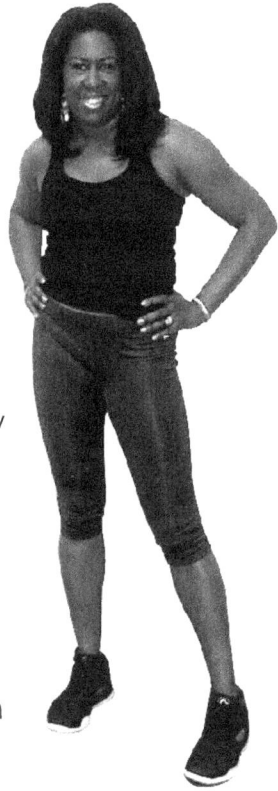

I have been a student my entire life; I have learned from many. If you read something in my book that sounds like something you may have heard elsewhere it is purely coincidental. The words in this book are my own.

**Don't Wait To Lose Weight**
**10 Steps to Kick-Start Your Fitness Journey**
Copyright © 2014 by Saideh Browne

ISBN: 978-0-9793642-2-8
Published by GS Publishing Group

This book is available at special discounts for churches, schools and other educational institutions.
Contact GS Publishing Group
201-263-4300

Author Bookings and Management
saidehbrowne@gmail.com

This book is dedicated to my five-am crew

# Your Fitness Success Map

Throughout the book you will see the following symbols; here are there meanings:

Stay Motivated

Get Moving

Meal Tip

# Prologue

Are you ready for the ride of your life? When I decided to lose weight I had no idea what to expect; and what actually happened I could have never expected. I don't want to scare you, really I don't, but you need to know *now* that losing weight is a journey. Honestly, your journey is not about losing weight, it's about realizing there are areas in your life that need to be addressed and how it's time for you to become committed to your personal success. My weight gain was the physical manifestation of my internal unhappiness. I found comfort in food and my body responded by increasing in size. Study after study details the evidenced-based connection between our mind and our body; there are intricately connected and are one. I knew I had to change.

As I began to remodel my reality I realized so many beliefs I once held true simply were not and my world of unicorns and rainbows slowly began to crumble. The beliefs I held so near and dear slowly evaporated into the ether. I watched people and things disappear; people and places and memories I wanted to hold onto I couldn't any longer. My life was changing.

I wanted to lose weight so badly I gave up old habits; I broke soul-ties and tossed the clutter (in every sense of the word). Purging was painful; but I'm much happier now because of it. Giving up old habits, breaking soul-ties and tossing clutter wasn't physically painful; the pain was derived from the mental fortitude needed to stay the course. The day I decided to lose weight was the day my realignment process began.

Making a decision to do anything is the best thing you can ever do for yourself. Make decisions swiftly and methodically and be prepared to live with the outcomes. Many times we ponder and wait and stew the process…that's a waste of time. Fear keeps us pondering. Why was I so afraid to lose weight? Upon reflection I realized I didn't want to face my food addiction and all the ugliness that came in that package. I said a prayer, made a decision and charged forward. "What's the worst that can happen, Saideh?" I thought, moments after becoming honest with myself. Maybe I'd look stupid in the gym. Maybe people would laugh at my struggle. Guess what! Those things happened and then some and I'm still standing. I don't look stupid in the gym anymore. People can't laugh at me because I'm not struggling like I was anymore and best of all I didn't fail.

The photo on the cover of this book was taken about 8 pounds heavier than my goal weight and I wasn't toned, but I redefined my reality and I made it happen on my terms. You're going to sweat, lose friends, cry, feel like crap, feel deflated, probably binge eat at some point, most likely try to starve yourself at some point but best of all you're going to get fit, change your life, forge ahead and motivate someone else. If I can do it, you can too.

Blessings

# Forward by Certified Personal Trainer Pamela Roundtree

Obesity in America is an epidemic. One in five children are obese with 300,000 being overweight. Heart disease is the number one killer in the United States according to the World Health Organization, yet we continue to grow outward. A few factors are at play here: our unhealthy addiction to sugar, the processed food we purchase and especially the unhealthy fast-food we consume. This is all exacerbated by our sedentary lifestyle – people just don't move as much as they used to.

Microwave ovens and Google have crippled us. Everyone is so impatient and we want everything right away; crash diets and appetite suppressant pills don't work over the long term and surgeries only marginally so. Obesity isn't something that happened to us in a month or even a year; those extra pounds developed slowly and methodically and the same approach is required to shed the excess weight – slowly and methodically. If being fit was easy, everyone would be fit and they're not. I help my clients stay motivated and encouraged to get fit daily. We set goals and we hit them as a team. Losing weight and becoming more fit and healthy is a challenge. I've been an athlete most of my life; in recent years I became lax with exercise and nutrition and in 2011 ballooned to 216 pounds; a weight I very uncomfortable with. The day after that sobering moment on the scale I joined the local gym. I started slowly. I went to the gym three times a week and changed my eating habits. Many of us work ten to twelve hours per day and cooking a healthy meal is the furthest thing from our thoughts but I made nutrition a priority in my life. I cut out fast foods, started cooking at home, preparing meals to take with me each day and I started reading food labels. One of the most important steps you can take to become healthier in life is to read and understand food labels; which will help you make better eating choices.

Food labels are required by the United States Food and Drug Administration for most prepared foods, such as breads, cereals, canned and frozen foods, snacks, desserts and drinks. For raw produce such as fruits and vegetables labeling is voluntary. I suggest you start by looking at the serving size and how many servings are in the package, this number is a point of reference for all of the other numbers on the label. For example; a frozen pizza may list 380 calories per serving and there are 4 servings in the box; that means if you eat the entire pizza at one sitting you are going to consume 1,520 calories! Food manufacturers are in the business of selling food, not making sure you're nutritionally aware of what you're eating. The onus, my friend, is on you.

The next step in properly reading and interpreting food labels is the daily value (DV) percentage. These numbers are of particular importance because they help you better factor the impact of consumption as it relates to your desired daily caloric and nutritional values intake. For example, based on your health needs you may need to consume extra iron, with that said a particular food item may only offer 10% of your daily iron intake per serving (based on a generic 2,000 calorie diet); that means you would need to consume 10 servings of that particular food item just to reach 100% of your daily recommended amount of iron. But, since your health plan requires additional iron you may need to consume an additional 5 servings to meet your goals. Here is the kicker. You will have now consumed 15 servings of this food item just to reach your recommended dosage of iron; but by consuming all of these servings you will have probably exceeded your recommended daily amounts of calories, sodium, fat and other nutrients. By understanding food labels you'll be able to easily discern what foods work and don't work with your body. We can all agree that the above sample food item is probably not the best source for your required daily iron intake. Reading and understanding food labels is so important but it goes hand in hand with understanding your body and what your body needs to function at an optimum level.

I salute your decision to lose weight and I leave you with insight and a few tips to help you understand some of the health claims food manufacturers make, along with a full-page infographic that explains food labels in more detail.

| | |
|---|---|
| Reduced | › Less than 25% of a specific nutrient |
| Good Source of | › 10% or more of a specific nutrient |
| High In | › 20% or more of a specific nutrient |
| Low Calorie | › 40 calories or less per serving |
| Calorie Free | › 5 calories or less per serving |
| Low Sodium | › 140mg of sodium or less per serving |

I wish you a NewMind.NewBody.NewLiving!

*Pamela Roundtree, Certified Personal Trainer*
*Owner, NewMind.NewBody.NewLiving*

# Learning to Read Food Labels

**Calories:** A calorie is a measure of energy use. Also listed is the number of calories from fat. The general rule is that no more than 30% of your calories should come from fat.

**% Daily Value:** This shows how much of the recommended amounts of these nutrients are in one serving (based on a 2,000 calorie diet). These percentages make it easy to compare one brand with another. Just make sure the serving size is the same. The goal is to eat no more than 100% of each nutrient each day.

**Vitamins & Minerals:** This shows you how much of the recommended amount of certain vitamins and minerals are in the food. Your goal is to reach 100% for each vitamin and mineral every day.

**Recommended Amounts:** Here you can see the recommended daily amount for each nutrient for 2 calorie levels: a 2,000 calorie and a 2,500 calorie daily diet. Your recommended daily calories may be higher or lower depending on your age, gender, and how active you are. However, notice that the recommended amount of sodium and cholesterol are the same no matter how many calories you eat a day.

Chicken Noodle Soup

## Nutrition Facts

Serving Size 1/2 cup (120 ml) condensed soup
Servings Per Container about 2.5

Amount Per Serving

| Calories 60 | Calories from Fat 15 |
| --- | --- |
| | % Daily Value* |
| **Total Fat** 1.5g | 2% |
| Saturated Fat 0.5g | 3% |
| Trans Fat 0g | |
| **Cholesterol** 15mg | 37% |
| **Sodium** 890mg | 3% |
| **Total Carbohydrate** 8g | 4% |
| Dietary Fiber 1g | |
| Sugars 1g | |
| **Protein** 3g | |

| Vitamin A | 4% | Calcium | 0% |
| --- | --- | --- | --- |
| Vitamin C | 0% | Iron | 2% |

*Percent Daily Values are based on a 2,000 calorie diet.
Your Daily Values may be higher or lower depending on your calorie needs.

| | Calories | 2000 | 2500 |
| --- | --- | --- | --- |
| Total Fat | Less than | 65g | 80g |
| Sat Fat | Less than | 20g | 25g |
| Cholesterol | Less than | 300mg | 300mg |
| Sodium | Less than | 2,400m | 2400mg |
| Total Carbohydrate | | 300g | 375g |
| Dietary Fiber | | 25g | 30g |

**Serving Size:** A serving size is usually less than most people eat. If you eat 2 servings, make sure you double the calories and all of the daily values. When comparing foods, make sure, the serving sizes are the same.

**Fat:** This lists the total amount of fat in one serving. Try to limit the amount of saturated fat and trans fat you eat.

**Cholesterol:** Try to eat less than 300 mg each day.

**Sodium:** Try to eat less than 2400 mg of sodium (salt) each day.

**Carbohydrates:** These help give you energy. They are found in bread, pasta, potatoes, fruits and vegetables. Good sources of fiber include fruits, vegetables, whole grains, and beans. Try to eat 20 to 35 g of fiber per day.

**Protein:** Protein helps build muscle. It is found in meat, nuts, eggs, fish, and dry beans. Try to eat lean cuts of meat.

Source: Adapted from: http://nutrition.about.com/od/recipesmenus/ss/learnlabels.htm

# CHAPTER ONE
## Your B.I.G. Decision

You are where you are because of who you were;
But where you go depends entirely on who you choose to be.
**Author Unknown**

Why is your life the way it is? Why are you where you are, doing what you're doing and living the way you're living? The answer is one word. Decisions. **Your personal power lies in your ability to make decisions.**

After graduating from college in 1996 I landed an amazing job in New York City working for a media company, I was 23 years old and making $25,000 per year ($40k in 2015). I had just given birth to my second son and felt as though my career and my life were on the right path. Since I was at the start of my career and worked long hours, my husband assumed many of the traditional mommy-duties, our roles were reversed long before "house-husband" was part of pop-culture lexicon. About a year into the position I told my boss I needed time off to take my children to the dentist; my 5 year old son for a basic checkup and my 1 year old son for a checkup and orthodontic assessment. He was a thumb sucker and we were concerned about the way his teeth were coming in. At three days old my little one carefully raised his thumb and it went right up his nose, then into both eyes and before long into his mouth. It was the cutest thing until his teeth started coming in. I knew we had to get ahead of this thing or be faced with a huge orthodontic bill in ten years. My boss granted my time off request and I took the kids to their appointment. While there the dentist advised that my younger son wasn't old enough to be seen by him and I needed to take him to another dental professional. "Cool," I thought and scheduled his appointment for the following week. The next morning I told my boss I needed to take an afternoon off the following week, he slightly slumped in his chair, inhaled slowly, exhaled even more slowly and said, "Ok." "What the hell?" I thought. My son was a year old, I rarely took time off, yet I was made to feel like shit because I needed to get my kid the necessary care to ensure a decent quality of life. I laughed (in my head) with disbelief. I walked back to my cubicle, slumped into my chair and at that very moment decided I will never, ever ask anyone permission to take care of my children. Ever!

That night I cried in my husband's arms. I asked him if I could quit and he said, "Yes." I went to work the very next day like nothing bothered me. My fascination with the inner workings of business increased while working for this media company and with a degree in Business Management I knew I wanted to work in a business environment, maybe something in operations or finance. A new Barnes and Noble bookstore had opened a half-block away from our office and I spent every lunch hour there for four months. I only cashed paychecks that were really, really needed to pay bills. And six months after that mortifying experience in my boss's office I quit my job. I had, what I thought, would be enough money to survive and I liberated myself.

I knew I needed money for living expenses but after scaling back for the past six months I knew my plan was doable. My salary was $25,000 per year which was $12.02 per hour before taxes; after taxes it comes to about $10.75 per hour. Now, remember I told you I was working in New York City, what I didn't share previously was that although I worked in the city, I lived in New Jersey which is quite common. This was problematic because I had to pay taxes to two different states. So that $10.75 per hour was actually about half-a-dollar less. Now, factor in transportation, dry cleaning, meals out because I worked late often and other expenses associated with two busy working parents and my actualized income was about $200 per week. So, I figured if I could run a business and earn about $200 per week I would actually be making the same amount of money and enjoy my children's childhood; some of which I missed because of college and work. My decision had been made and now had to figure out what life was going to look like as a 26 year old self-employed mom with a two year old and a six year old. Remember, this was in the late 90's; this lifestyle was an anomaly. I remember my grandmother asking me earnestly, "Saideh, what am I going to tell the people in church what you do for a living?" I told her to tell them, "I work every day, just like they do."

The decision to quit my job changed the trajectory of my life. I was out of the workforce and had to figure out how to feed my family, pay bills, pay for the children's education and manage to stay sane. I received so much backlash because of my decision, it was brutal. I heard, "What are you going to do about your 401k?" "How are you going to make it?" "What are you going to put on your resume if you have to go back to work?" See, all of those questions, I felt, would answer themselves because the reason I quit was because to become a mom; something that is not shameful nor something to be embarrassed over. I practiced my canned responses, with the most popular likening my life to those mom's in the 50's whose husbands worked while they stayed home and tended to the house. Sometimes I was met with resistance ever after my explanation. I remember thinking why did I even had to justify my life to anyone, I realized then I was different. Now, here we are almost 25 years later and many people want to quit their jobs to become their own boss; I laugh because I had a huge head start and part of my income now is derived from consulting the very people who doubted me. My children are better off because I was home with them; they saw me hustle, run several businesses over the years and I am still married. Things worked out for the best.

Making tough decisions is never easy, especially if people don't see what you see. It's lonely, it's scary and sometimes it's hard for you to even comprehend why you made the decision you did in the first place. But, hear me though, trust your own voice. I cannot even count the number of times where my own self-doubt slowed me down; but I stayed the course. I've only had four real jobs my entire adult life and each of these positions were taken at pivotal moments; my younger son started school; my older son started middle school; my younger son graduated from high school and as each of these pivotal moments played out I assessed my life and felt out of place and out of touch with my peers. I suffered from depression for a while because I felt, momentarily, that I was missing out on something − life even.

None of those jobs ever lasted very long. I always came back to my *why.* My why was to be a mom and even though I felt left out of society at times my spirit was at peace taking care of my family.

Ask anyone, male or female, who is a minute from turning 40 years old and they will all tell you the same thing, "I need to get my life together." Socioeconomic status doesn't matter in this case, everyone is equal; gender doesn't even matter. Everyone sobers up when they approach that special birthday and I was no different. To celebrate the occasion my husband and I took a much-needed trip to Jamaica and when we got back home and really looked at the pictures I realized I was fat, and that feeling sucked. I was fat and didn't know what to do about it. No one saw it but me. But then again, that's the story of my life. I often see in myself what others don't see – all of my super powers and all of my vulnerabilities. I joined a local gym and began my fitness journey. Never in a million years would I imagine that I'd become a fitness professional. But that's the real beauty in living your truth. It's your truth even if no one else sees it.

I made several decisions in my life; the three biggest being having a child at 18, having a second child at 22 and quitting my job at 23. We can all agree that perhaps had these decisions not been made I would have gone to an "away-school" instead of "staying local." Perhaps I'd be the CEO of that media company now if I had never quit; but one thing is for sure I set goals for myself and I worked every day to achieve them. My first goal was to make $200 per week; done. My second goal was to make enough money to raise happy, balanced children; done. My next goal in life was to lose weight; that goal was the hardest to design and the most difficult to work through. At this point in my life it wasn't just about setting a goal and smashing it, it was about setting a goal and breaking 35 years of habits. Our habits form as a child when our parents set the tone of what is and is not acceptable. My earlier goals were easy and simple because no precedence had been set; this weight loss and healthy eating thing was a totally different story.

⭐ Start a life of health and fitness today, not tomorrow and certainly not on Monday

Healthy eating means different things to many people, and everyone assumes it's one thing or another based on their perspectives and relationships; **healthy eating is simply eating in a way that optimizes *your* health.** For example, my body may need extra fiber so healthy eating for me may consist of bran infused breads; whereas your body may require extra calcium so healthy eating for you may consist of salmon three times a week. No meal plan is a catch all for everybody. There are, of course, certain meal plans that blanket populations under certain circumstances. For example, nursing moms will certainly require additional nutrients regardless of height, weight, body fat percentage or geographic location, which is a fact. Your new life of health and fitness is not a temporary change; rather a massive fundamental shift in your being. Start small so you can actualize your progress; make it something you can live with daily and chart your progress day in and day out.

Many fitness professionals believe that before starting any health program you should consult a doctor; I don't. I believe when you feel you're ready to change your life you should just start – right then and right there. It's too easy to find reasons to kick the can down the road; setting an appointment, keeping the appointment and following through adds too many layers and points where procrastination can occur. You'll know when you're ready, and when you're ready just start. Your spirit will guide you on where to begin. In the beginning, trust your spirit and let it guide you. It knows exactly what to do. As a result of your intention the world will respond in kind. People will make suggestions and offer tips to help you out and even make recommendations of good books to read (like this one ☺). Then, when you're really ready, you'll consult with your doctor, meet with a nutritionist and start working with a personal trainer because you made a spiritual decision and you're ready for powerful results. You know what your *why* is and your *why* will lead you down the right path and into the hands of professionals who will support you. And guess what? You'll do exactly what you have to do because you want it so badly. You'll work successfully without coercion and force. Starting is the most difficult aspect of developing and maintaining a healthy lifestyle, but once you do success becomes attainable.

You'll soon learn the basic tenets of health and fitness are all the same; with the most important being eating less harmful foods and eating more helpful foods. Yes, my formula is oversimplified but it's really the truth. Temptation is all around us and I didn't even realize I had a food addiction until I hired a weight loss coach. She helped me see that I ate for every reason in the book except for nutrition! I consciously made healthier foods more appealing than unhealthy ones and mentally connected unhealthy foods to the way I was and connected healthy foods to my future.

Eating better was literally moment by moment decisions because I was eating for no reason throughout the day.

Making a radical change in my life probably would have been easier but I knew a crash diet wasn't sustainable over the long haul. I started with cutting the skin off of chicken thighs and legs; eventually I stopped eating thighs and legs and enjoyed lean cuts of chicken breasts and tenders; the result was a tremendous reduction of fat in my mid-section which led to a reduction in my overall body fat percentage. Don't overlook the importance of small changes.

Replace whole milk with skim or 2% both for drinking and in recipes

Snack on low fat frozen yogurt instead of ice cream

Spray pans with non-fat cooking spray instead of butter or margarine

Eat more fish and less red meat

Use egg whites and substitutes for eating and cooking

There are so many other tips I will share in this book and online at saidehbrowne.com to help you move forward and create significant health improvements in your life no matter what your goal is right now. Your goals will change over time but today is the day to start the rest of your life. No matter what your current level of health is, eating a healthier diet and losing weight guarantees you a better quality of life in your later years. Think of this as a marathon and not a sprint. The goal of any healthy eating program is to make lifestyle changes, how you prepare your meals, the way you grocery shop and where you dine out that leads to life-long success.

Your B.I.G. Decision today is to **B**elieve **I**n your **G**oals.

My Goals are:

_____

_____

_____

_____

_____

_____

_____

_____

_____

_____

# Chapter Two
## Create A Plan

Failing to plan is planning to fail.
**Alan Lakein, Acclaimed Time Management Author**

Do you want me to guarantee your success? I can you know. Really, I can. But first you need to create a plan; and the success of this plan hinges upon two character traits that must be more fervently developed at this time in your life. They are discipline and commitment. **Discipline** involves planning and execution. **Commitment** guarantees your ability to stay in the game long enough to reach your goal. Many people plan things but what's lacking is the ability to focus and the lack of persistence and tenacity. These traits are particularly challenging to master for creative people like me; I, like many others, work best when our spirit moves. This is a guaranteed route to failure when the need arises to accomplish a specific goal. This book, for example, was planned in my head for a year and then drafted on paper here and there over the course of another year but it wasn't until a tiny spark caught fire that I was able to knock this book out over a long weekend. I didn't have a plan for this book and as a result it took too long to publish. Why was I able to knock this book out in a weekend when all of my previous attempts produced no fruit? Because, the discipline and commitment to the process and end result simply wasn't there. When I wanted this book completed badly enough it miraculously got done. Did I want it done sooner? Of course; but what I felt like doing (everything but writing this book) superseded what I needed to do (write this book) and as a result my goal (publishing this book) never manifested (under my old strategies). This book was delayed because I wasn't disciplined and committed enough to make it happen. Once my spark was ignited I created my massive action plan, and voilà you're reading my 7$^{th}$ book.

⭐ A goal without a plan is just a wish

Your weight loss goal, no matter the amount of weight you want to lose, must contain three components:
1.  Meals
2.  Movement
3.  Motivation

From this moment on, decide to be driven by your goals and not your past. Let the past remain in the past – let it be gone forever. Now is the time to chart new waters with a new compass. You can become whatever it is you want to become and you can look however you want to look once you're disciplined and committed. Your plan is really your written design for your future. Yes, this book is about losing weight but it's secretly about helping you achieve success in every area of your life. Live your life according to your plan and you will become the person you've been dreaming about. You've investing so much time and energy into everything that hasn't worked, or worked only marginally so; those days are over. No more wavering dreams, no more long unfulfilled to-do lists see your future as you want and achieve it. This is the beginning of your new you. It is now and forever about achieving success in every area of your life starting with your health and being fit. From today on you will grow and move forward in a profound, meaningful and dramatic way because you choose to. I know you will accomplish your goals. How do I know? Because you are going to create a plan and you're going to be disciplined and committed enough to get where you want to be. I believe in you. Do you believe in yourself?

Success is within your reach because you're now tapping the surface of your unlimited power and potential. Being healthy and fit is the only option for your life right now. Being overweight and unhealthy is in your past; that's the old you. The new you purchased this book and is ready to live again! Have confidence in yourself, believe you can do it and you will. Connect with others who will challenge you, it hurts but it will make you grow. I stopped counting how many times I cursed my trainer in my head. I remember on one of my 5am training days he had me deadlifting (a strength training exercise where I take a deep squat then stand straight up while lifting a barbell with heavy weights on both ends) with a count of 15 repetitions three times; I knocked the first two out the box and by the third set I tiredly looked up and asked if I could stop at 10 and he stared matter-of factly back at me and quietly said, "Fifteen." I wanted to cry but I made it to 15. He challenged me and still does. I actually didn't like the accountability at first because it was something I wasn't used to. I didn't like the text messages and the constant checking in but now I totally understand that is exactly what I needed to get from where I was to where I wanted to be; he became an integral part of my plan.

## Chapter Two / Part Two
## Meal Planning

When it comes to losing weight, your diet (meaning what you eat and not an actual meal plan) and movement are the two most critical components; with diet being more important than movement. When I first started the journey I would take two group fitness classes each morning and for lunch eat an entire oven baked pizza; I'd go back to the gym at night and eat fried chicken with macaroni and cheese and collard greens for dinner. This went on for weeks and I couldn't understand why I wasn't losing weight. I rationalized that the gym was scamming me and I wanted to quit. Oliver Wendell Holmes, Jr. famously said, "A mind that is stretched by a new experience can never go back to its old dimensions," and this was my predicament. After a few weeks in the gym and about one-hundred group fitness classes under my belt I realized, maybe the gym wasn't scamming me, maybe something needed to change on my end. I became chatty with some gym ladies and began networking in the sauna and each of these conversations fed me a little piece here and a little piece there and soon realized I would never be able to outwork a bad diet. I could work out all day but appetizers and drinks with the girls at night would set me back more calories than I burned in the gym all day. What a sobering revelation. But guess what was happening? I was beginning to grow. I slowed down happy-hour with the girls, I ate less calories during the day and I stopped eating after

8pm. As I grew that wasn't enough, I wanted more; I needed more and I started paying attention to my triggers one of which was fast and easy food. The low cost of wings at happy-hour, a Whopper Jr. from Burger King or a junior cheeseburger deluxe from Wendy's made it too easy for me to pit-stop at the drive-thru and knock down a quick 700 calories. Do you know how long it takes to burn 700 calories on a treadmill? Yeah, for me, in those days about 50 minutes. I knew I had to start preparing my food or else I'd never stop eating junk food on the go.

The first thing I decided to do was not eat out for a week and that meant I'd have to have, at-the-ready, something on hand whenever I needed to eat. This forced me to prepare, in advance, a morning snack, lunch and an afternoon snack. I headed to the store and this is what I bought:

- ✓ Plastic containers with a tight lid
- ✓ Case of water
- ✓ Lemons and limes
- ✓ Family size package of chicken breast
- ✓ Big bag of frozen tilapia
- ✓ Package of frozen salmon
- ✓ Frozen package of small ears of corn
- ✓ Bag of frozen green beans
- ✓ Package of Rice cakes
- ✓ Bag of potatoes
- ✓ Celery
- ✓ 3 Medium size tomatoes
- ✓ Square napkins
- ✓ Tub of powdered protein mix
- ✓ Package of napkins

The next day I cooked all of the fish I bought, all of the chicken I bought, all of the potatoes I bought and all of the corn and green beans I bought. Once all of this food was cooked − and it was a lot of food − I began packaging it. I mixed and matched all of the food items so no two containers were the same and I portion controlled the sizes to make sure I wasn't overeating.

Meat    › 3 ounces is the about the size of your palm
Veggies › A portion is about the size of your fist
Starch   › A little smaller than the size of your fist

Once all of the containers were packed I left them on the counter to cool. I put three of them in the refrigerator and the rest into the freezer. It seemed like I spent a lot of money at the grocery store but in all actuality I had enough packaged meals to last almost two workweeks. The following week I purchased:

- ✓ Ground turkey
- ✓ Mozzarella cheese
- ✓ Pasta sauce
- ✓ A bag of baby spinach
- ✓ Little packages of non-fat salad dressing
- ✓ An avocado
- ✓ A box of protein bars
- ✓ Yogurt and sugar-free pudding

The next day I made a huge pan of baked ziti and once it cooled I packaged it into containers as well. By now my freezer was stocked with packaged foods I prepared lovingly for my body from my kitchen. I lowered the salt intake on all of the recipes and made sure I used spices that contained little or no sugar in the ingredients, you'd be surprised by how many over the counter seasonings contain sugar.

During that past week and for the next few weeks I didn't eat fast food for lunch – which saved a ton of money – and I ate much, much healthier. It became pleasurable picking out what I was going to eat for lunch each night before I went to bed. I'd peruse my freezer, take a container of food out and place it on the kitchen counter; by the time I woke up the next morning my lunch for the day was thawed. My system was so effective that my husband joined in and started taking my lunch packages for his lunch as well ☺.

Soon after, we increased food production and used the extra meals for dinner. Food prep, as I call it, it not as laborious as it may seem; the key is overcooking food when you are in the kitchen cooking. This way you're not in the kitchen everyday trying to find something to eat and subsequently eating bad food late at night; a double whammy to your diet. As far as snacks go, I love rice cakes and those are super easy to toss in my bag; I suggest once you open the package to put the remaining rice cakes into a Ziploc bag because, to me, they get stale after about a week. I also love celery, so I cut up celery stalks and put them in small bags so I can eat them on the go, forgo ranch or bleu cheese dip. I love crunchy foods so my challenge is to find alternative crunchy foods that I can eat on the go that are not chips, pretzels and bad carbohydrates.

Preparing meals in advance helps you stay disciplined to your goal and makes commitment easier. I'm all about easier. Listen, life is always going to throw us curve balls and things are going to pop up but preparing your meals in advance helps to control this area of your life where you may be the most vulnerable. This system works not matter how many kids you have to shuttle to dance class or soccer practice or how late you have to work to finish a major report due for your boss. You now have a strategy to tackle the most challenging aspect of your weight loss journey and that's eating unhealthy foods.

I encourage you to keep a good supply of sugar-free pudding, yogurt, fruits and salad ingredients on hand at all times. A salad is a great way to produce a well-rounded meal quite quickly. If you start with arugula or fresh baby spinach you can add walnuts, raisins, cranberries and other sweet fruits to your base then add egg, tuna, grilled chicken or another protein and top it off with a light vinaigrette. You'll satisfy your taste buds and still eat clean. It's important to resist the temptation to raid the fridge late at night; already having something to eat takes the guess work out of your day, which actually frees up more time for you to better enjoy the things and people you love the most.  High calorie packaged foods are a killer in every sense of the word; don't let them win! Food manufacturers are banking on your weakness and unpreparedness, why give them the satisfaction of higher profits at your expense. As a last resort and when you're in a pinch, you can even purchase a few meals designed for dieters located in the frozen section of your local grocery store. This isn't what I'd like for you because of the high sodium content of these meals along with many other reasons, but this is a better alternative to eating from a drive-thru.

I realize you cannot pack and take your food with you for the rest of your life; lunch and dinner invitations are inevitable and you'll need coping strategies for those moments too. I'm a media entrepreneur in the top media market of the world and in one of the busiest cities in the world and I'm invited to lunches a lot and evening networking events and cocktail receptions even more. I forced myself to develop ways to navigate those moments where I'm asked to attend an event and all I really want to do is go home and eat a salad. Luckily most places in New York City offer low calorie meals and healthy alternatives so I try to redirect evening meetings and business opportunities to mid-day but some events like album release parties, venue openings, fashion shows and other affairs only happen during dinner hours. First, if it's a sit down dinner I order a salad instead of an appetizer; for the main course I go for chicken or a light flaky fish and I steer clear of any bread or pasta especially if I had a portion of carbs during the day. Then, once my food arrives I immediately (and immediately is the key) request a take-home container and by the time I bless my food the server has returned with a portable container. I carefully portion my entrée in half and place one entire half of whatever I ordered into the to-go container. This has been a winning strategy for me because it prevents me from a) overeating b) picking over my food once I'm full c) allows me to focus on the dinner conversation to get the deal done versus shoveling food down my throat all night. This works for me and I know it can work for you.

Lastly, understand that everyone is not going to be happy for you. They may say they are but they really are not. This is how I know. My friends kept asking me to go out to happy-hour and for drinks on Friday's and after I declined gracefully several times, they even offered to pay my tab! This will happen to you. It's not that your friends don't want you to lose weight per se, but they see your weight loss as a reminder of their inability to be disciplined and commit to their goals. I saw this first-hand and it really hurt; and it hurt even more coming from my closest friends. I started this journey around my 40th birthday and by that time in my life many of my friends were slightly (but bearably) overweight, settled in their careers, married with kids in high school – maybe middle school and had no real reason to get fit. So subconsciously their kindness was really sabotage to my goals. I can't stress how much this pained me once I realized what was going on, but it made me stronger and made me more determined to lose weight and become healthier. Once they saw my unwillingness to deter from my goals they backed off, the invites came less frequently and I felt alone. Here's the best part though, I only felt alone for a little while because where I lost unhealthy friends, I gained a boatload of new friends who only wanted to see me happy on my journey. Isn't that amazing! My new friends and I ate out more frequently than I did with my other friends but we ate at vegan restaurants, we ate egg whites when we all went out for brunch and we did, on occasion, enjoy a mimosa or two. The difference was they supported me and I needed that. I needed people around me who weren't going to question why I peeled the skin off the chicken or why I ate a double dose of broccoli instead of a veggie and a starch with my entrée. I needed the extra love and support because everything was so new to me at the time. Trust your plan and daringly move forward, no matter what. When they're ready you'll be the head of the inaugural support team they'll need.

## Chapter Two / Part Three
## Movement

Being active helps you live healthy and strong and isn't that what we all want? Exercise and fitness are not just for people who have weight issues, having full range of motion and being able to move your limbs freely has more benefits that I would ever be able to list in this book. Exercise and movement mean different things to different people; for me it's about the weight loss, for my husband it's about building his upper body and for my children it's about them being limber on the basketball court. In 2012 I was attending a week-long conference in New York City and getting around that town in a vehicle is no easy fete, so in the interest of time I walked everywhere. I was still relatively new on my fitness journey but my health and agility had drastically improved. By Wednesday, mid-week of the conference I began to feel a sharp pain in my side, I chalked it up to gas and kept my day going. On Thursday, the pain in my side kept recurring, I knew then it wasn't gas but I figured it was something I ate from a vending truck that didn't agree with me. By the last day of the conference I was in excruciating pain and I knew something was wrong. I was in so much pain that morning I decided to drive to the conference because I wasn't able to get around very well. Thankfully, since it was the last day of the conference all activities ended at 12 noon. As soon as the conference was over I planned on driving to the emergency room but I couldn't make it. I drove to the office where I do a lot of charity work and the team there called my husband and then an ambulance. By the time my husband arrived at the hospital they had me under observation and had administered pain medication; which didn't help much. They ran test after test for hours and nothing showed up. My mom lost a courageous battle with ovarian cancer just three years prior so some type of cancer or cyst or problem with any of my female moving parts was not ruled out. By early evening they diagnosed me with an appendix that was about to rupture. I had been walking around with an appendix that could have ruptured at any moment for three days. They scheduled my surgery for the next available time slot. Unfortunately a gunshot victim was brought into the hospital so my surgery was bumped from late that night to first thing in the morning. I was scared and hungry and in severe pain.

When they called me for surgery I was ready, the pain was severe and my husband was still by my side. The ebbs and flow of pain prevented me from getting any modicum of sleep; I wanted the pain to be gone. I awakened in the recovery room and was still in pain. Soon, the nurses brought in my husband. He was by my side when I needed him the most. When I was wheeled up to my room I was greeted by two close friends; one had brought me a satin pillowcase (she said hospital pillow cases would wreak havoc on my hair) and the other brought a warm smile and her adorable six-year old daughter. I was happy because they were there and more so because I was no longer in excruciating pain.

On discharge day I was told I'd be out of commission for a minimum of four weeks and probably closer to six weeks – that meant no gym and no major physical exertion; I was devastated. After playing games during the first six months of my fitness journey I had finally hit a good stride with my meals and workouts and now I was sidelined. I was devastated. During the first week of my recovery I had plenty of visitors. I left my front door open so company could stroll in; I needed that. I needed to see I wasn't a cripple and out of people's hearts and minds. By the end of the first week I was up walking, I felt great and was really getting around the house. One of my friends accompanied me to the doctor for my two-week post-operative appointment, I insisted on driving. My surgeon gave me great news, I was progressing well and healing much better than he expected. I asked if I could go back to the gym and his long paused led me to believe he was going to tell me no, but he didn't. He told me I could go back to the gym and resume working out if I felt up to it. Hell yeah! I felt up to it! Cabin fever was beginning to set in anyway and I needed to get out of the house. By the end of week two I resumed yoga and by the beginning of week four I was back into my full-body work outs and this time I was super determined to make every work out count. Being told I couldn't work out was a sharp pin that pierced my balloon. I never appreciated working out so much until I was told I couldn't do so. I went in hard and never looked back. During my two week follow up appointment my surgeon told me, as I was walking out the door, that I was

41

able to recover so quickly because I was in good shape. You don't know how good I felt hearing that from a stranger. His compliment meant more to me than hearing from any of my old friends or even my husband for that matter. He greenlit my early return to the gym because my body was the physical manifestation of all the work I had put in. I could have jumped over the moon that day. Could I have recovered successfully had I not been in good shape? Of course. Would my recovery had been as speedy? Probably not. I know exercise works!

K Mild to moderate exercising is:

  a) an easy way to improve overall health
  b) a way to extend our lives
  c) a great way to feel happier

My exercise regimen, when I first started out, included group fitness classes at a local gym and power walks and light jogs on the treadmill. Your program will likely not resemble what mine looks like now, but in the beginning I suggest you start where I did. Check out your local community center to see if there are free or low-cost classes you can take, this is a safe and welcoming place to start. I suggest starting with group classes because it's a great segue to relationships with other's on the journey.

K If exercising in a facility is not for you then try these:

1. Take a 30 minute walk in your neighborhood or around your local park. This is an effective way to bond with your children, your partner and close friends. If 30 minutes is too much then start with 15 minutes, 2 to 3 days per

week. You can increase the duration of your walks as your body builds endurance.

2. Include your family in your fitness life and workout routine. If they're the ones holding you back then govern yourself accordingly; but if they're supportive keep them close by. Honor your time with them and respect that yes, they may support your decision to lose weight but they don't want to be alienated in the process. If you plan your workouts during family obligations you're setting yourself up for failure. Find out what time blocks you can control (such as waking up earlier) and use that time to plan your work outs.

3. Join a fitness program at work. If your job doesn't have one, why don't you start one? Talk with your boss and get something going with your immediate peers and colleagues. This is what my husband did. He started working out during his lunch break and after a while a few guys joined him. Of course they're not doing a major, intense full-body workout but they do squats, lunges, jumping jacks and other low intensity calisthenics.

4. Exercise while cleaning the house and performing other household chores. I can attest that gardening in the spring, raking leaves in the fall and shoveling snow burns a ton of calories.

5. Go bowling, roller-skating, snow tubing or some other 2-3 person activity. These are low cost − high calorie burning activities that rev up your heart rate, speeds your metabolism and burns fat quickly.

These activities can burn from 150 to 1,000 calories per session! That's a lot of calories. When you're working out your body produces and releases endorphins. Endorphins diminish the perception of pain thereby altering your mood to make you feel better. This is why people who exercise are smiling and happy even after the most grueling workout. Good workouts partnered with good nutrition will make you feel better and give you a rosier outlook on life.

If all of these are still tough for you, try working fitness into your day, instead of stopping your day for fitness. You can take the stairs instead of the elevator; park your car further from the door or even use your arms and legs more when carrying groceries in the house. There are several neat things you can do to trick your body once your fitness goals are established and you're disciplined and committed. What I don't want you to do is overexert yourself. Don't ever, ever force your body a few degrees past what's is capable of at this point on your journey; one day on and one day off is a great schedule to follow in the beginning. If you get hurt, stop immediately and seek medical attention. Be smart about accomplishing your goals. I learned what my limits were and I didn't care how fast or agile everybody else in the class was I kept my own pace. Remember when I shared with you the story of my appendectomy? Well, when I returned to yoga class no one knew I had just had surgery; imagine if I tried to pick up where I had left off two weeks prior. I would have delayed full recovery just to prove to everyone in the class that I still had "it," when I really didn't. I was recovering from surgery and I had to keep reminding myself of that with each movement I cut short for fear of injuring myself. You didn't get to where you are in a day or even a week for that matter, so take it easy and do the best you can every single day. Once you give your body time to adjust to your new fitness routine, your sleep will improve and you will experience more clarity in all other areas of your life.

## Chapter Two / Part Four
## Motivation

Weight loss success is measured, by most, in numbers. "How much weight have you lost?" "What is your body fat percentage now?" "How long has it taken you to lose the weight?" "What size are you now?" "How much weight do you want to lose?" I can go on and on; but what cannot be measured by numbers is your happiness with yourself. This is 100% personal and 100% all you. If you want to reach your weight loss goal then you already know you have to watch what you eat and exercise; but the $3^{rd}$ ingredient is the right attitude. A few pages ago I shared with you how I felt when I began losing friends because of my weight loss, then in the sentences immediately after I raved about all of the new friends I acquired; this is a peek into your journey in the near future. It's filled with highs and lows. Use this time in your life to uncover undiscovered opportunities to live to your highest potential. Do things you've never done before...live a little. Good things are bound to happen if you allow them to.

At one point in my adult life my husband and I along with our two sons moved into my grandmother's home. My grandfather had passed and she really didn't need to live by herself anymore. We sold our house and moved into hers.

Emotionally this was tough, we sold everything we owned because she had everything in her house already. We didn't even need to bring our beds. We sold our furniture, pots, dishes, washing machine, I mean damn near everything. Move in day wasn't the joyous, celebratory experience I thought it would be; we moved our clothes in and shoved a few personal items into a corner in the basement and that was that. A few months into our new living arrangements, arguments ensued. Nothing major in the beginning, but heightened enough; coupled with our shared feelings of separation from our belongings created what would become a simmering pot ready to boil over at any moment.

Not every day was dipped in doubt – we enjoyed some wonderful Sunday dinners and insightful moments just sitting on the porch listening to her stories of slavery, the Great Depression, the Civil Rights Movement, the death of Martin Luther King, the death of my grandfather from her perspective and her hopes and dreams for my small family. As of this writing, my grandmother is 94 years old and I can't imagine what my life would be like had I not spent five wonderful years in her space, enjoying her company, feeling her presence and understanding her love. Motivation is not about a man on a stage telling you how crappy your life is then hawking products to make you feel better; nor is it attending Sunday worship service singing and dancing like David yet leaving the sanctuary unfulfilled by the leader's message. What motivates you is 100% personal and 100% all you. This book swirled in my head for a year then spent another year doodled on scraps of paper in unfinished sentences; the motivation to get this book published was not external; it was internal. Something inside me said, "It's time," and I followed my spirit's lead.

**Be bold and industrious.** I heard motivational speaker Tony Robbins say, "Failure is not due to lack of resources, but lack of resourcefulness." I challenge you to be resourceful and hardworking, never stop looking ahead and never lose focus of why you started this journey in the first place. Work harder than anybody else, stay up late and do 10 pushups, delay the gratification of that bowl of ice-cream until you lose one more pound. Change your schedule if need be to accommodate your new workout routine. Keep a list of people on hand who can pick up the kids in case you're running late from the gym. Do whatever you have to do to make this thing work. You got this!

**Be resilient.** Everyone has problems; are you going to let them stop you or just temporarily slow you down? Fail fast, learn from your mistakes and improve on your systems as you learn. Give yourself a few minutes to grieve, cry, sulk and pout then pick yourself up and be doubly determined to make it the next time. Many of the most successful people failed miserably before they made it. Why are you any different? Set realistic expectations and enjoy the journey.

**Be forever hopeful.** Stay positive about any and every situation in your life. I know it may be difficult when you're in it but trust me, there is always light at the end of the tunnel. I heard popular televangelist Joyce Myer once say, "…you're only going through. In the good times and the bad times, you're only going through." She's right! When good times are a-rollin' remember they won't last forever; and when bad times have you down remember they won't last forever either. Be optimistic and encouraged in all that you do. The more you smile the more the world will smile back at you. Set your intention on new opportunities and new people and I guarantee new opportunities and new people will find you. The question is, "Will you be ready to receive everything coming your way?" Be ready so you don't have to get ready.

**Be patient.** Some of your goals may be super-big and cannot be accomplished in a month or even three months. Great things take time. Don't be afraid to dream big because accomplishing your goals may take a long time, wait it out. Use all of the minutes in your day to *be ready* so as you inch closer to your personal goals you don't have to *get ready.* Patience is an acquired skill; success is measured not by how many times you fall, but by how many times you rise.

**Do this for yourself.** So many people start living a healthy life because they have to, not because they want to. Winston Churchill has said, "Americans will always do what's right, once they have exhausted all other alternatives." Make your journey the *only* option − resist other alternatives and short cuts. Lovers may come and go and impressing a potential partner is good reason to get your life together, but it shouldn't be the prevailing reason. Any reason, outside of doing this for yourself, is not reason enough to keep you committed; as soon as those reasons are no longer important in your life your journey won't be important in your life either. Do this to make your life better, you don't need anyone's approval to validate how great you are. After all, the only approval you'll ever need is your own.

# Chapter Three
## Get A Partner

Each person holds so much power within themselves that needs to
be let out. Sometimes they just need a little nudge, a little direction,
a little support, a little coaching and the greatest things can happen.
**Pete Carroll, Professional Football Coach**


When I joined the gym they offered me a tour of their
facility and showed me a list of their classes, I didn't care how
nice they were I was so overwhelmed. Thankfully, I was
assured that everyone felt like I did that day. I was comforted
somewhat. I was far too intimidated to get on any of the
machines so I took a group fitness class and stood in the
back by the door. After a few classes, I gained some
confidence but I still stood in the back. One morning the
club manager stopped me and asked me how everything was
going? I told him I was still a bit lost but I was getting there.
He offered me a complimentary personal training session with
one of the trainers and I accepted. The session was brutal I
tell you, just brutal. I didn't realize how out of shape I was. It
was bad. Of course, after the session, the trainer wanted to
sign me on as a client and I gracefully declined. "They're not
going to scam me," I thought. I continued in the gym doing
what I thought was right and what I felt comfortable doing.

A few months later the gym introduced a weight loss program that guaranteed I'd lose up to 28 pounds during my first month on the program; it took some convincing but I signed a two year agreement for the program; it was one the best decisions I've made in my life. I always thought the gym was trying to scam me – hey, I'm from New York and we're suspicious of everybody; but they were just trying to help me. Yes, the gym needs to make money and a profit but their staff genuinely wanted to help me lose weight. The program provided a weight loss coach, food-shopping lists, face-to-face coaching and many other benefits; it was amazing. After working with a coach for almost a year, I hit my goal weight! My weight loss coach and I became friends and there is no way in the world I would have hit my goal weight without her. She was the partner I needed. **Everyone needs a change partner;** someone who can listen, hear you, have empathy, chastise you when necessary and keep you committed to why you started this journey in the first place.

When my two-year contract was almost up, I signed on for personal training; another great decision on my part. There is no way I could have gotten my body into the shape it is in now without a trainer. There is so much information on the web and in bookstores but all of the information out there is generalized. My weight loss coach and personal trainer worked with me and for me to create a coordinated program designed for my body type and eating habits, which made my effort much more targeted and effective.

Having a coach and a trainer was never in my budget but I made it work. I am not some rich housewife who spends

50

her husband's money with reckless abandon, I am a typical middle age women who works everyday like many others. The money appeared once I became 100% committed to my personal success. I cut a few things out and shaved some things here and there but the biggest infusion of cash came from the most unexpected line item in my budget – my weekly grocery bill. I swear, once I stopped purchasing junk food I had almost $60 per week extra in my budget. At this point in my life my older son was living on his own, my younger son had just graduated from high school; he was still at home but was always out with friends so I was really just purchasing food for my husband and I. I did not realize how much I would spend for a typical Friday movie night at home; Pillsbury cookies $4.95 for the big log; two frozen pizza's $5.95 each; a gallon of iced tea $3.75; three pints of ice cream at $3.85 each totals $28.30! That's thirty bucks out and 2,000 calories in, now multiply that by four Friday's in a month; that $120 is exactly one and a half times what I was paying for my weight loss coach each month. You can do this. Where there is will, there is away.

If having a personal trainer and weight loss coach is not feasible for you right now, for whatever reason, look for an online program. So many online programs are convenient and cost less than a face-to-face program like the one I had – some are even free and can connect with your mobile device. If you are on Facebook do a search for weight loss groups, there are many to choose from; join one and utilize the friendships you form in the group as your support system. My challenge to you is to get a partner...somehow. You don't have to do this alone. Everyone needs a friend and this is a tough road to go alone. Having a supportive ear and an ally makes it more bearable.

# Chapter Four
# Get Moving

*If a man achieves victory over his body,*
*who in the world can exercise power over him?*
**Vinoba Bhave, Indian Advocate of Nonviolence and Human Rights**

As you'll learn on your path to losing weight, effective weight loss is not only about watching what you eat, but much more about challenging and changing your current lifestyle. This means changing your habits and how you navigate your daily life. All of us at some point may feel sad, alone and down in the dumps, and that's normal but if we stay in that place too long we may become chronically depressed. When our body is in motion— either by everyday activities or in an actual workout endorphins are released which are known to block the sensation of pain and make you feel better. Don't you want to feel good and not depressed? Then, get moving!

One morning, on my way to the gym, the lid detached from my coffee cup as I was placing it into the cup holder in the armrest of my car. Not only did I spill piping hot coffee on my lap but it was all over the armrest and on my seat. I didn't have enough time to clean it up before my class was scheduled to start so I took my sweat towel and used that to dry up my seat and soak up some of the coffee in the arm est. I loathe the smell of coffee (unless I'm drinking it) and I keep a spotless car so this really pissed me off. As I was driving, I asked the Universe aloud, "I hope this is not indicative of my day?" I dashed to the gym and my class hadn't started yet so I jumped on the scale; the numbers fluttered and settled on 176.6. "What the hell?" I thought. I smelled like stale coffee, my car seat was soaked from spilled coffee, I had no towel to dry off during class and I weighed a few more pounds than the last time I jumped on the scale. I felt screwed and it was only six minutes after five in the morning!

Something happened during my work out that morning, I cried. The more I worked out the more I cried. Tears flowed as I worked out all of the emotions that swelled within the past hour. Sometimes the gym is my church and the workout is my moment at the altar. Moving past boundaries and breaking chains is empowering. I was so moved during those sacred moments that the emotional tone had been set for the rest of my day – nothing and I mean nothing was going to tear me down. I was invincible. During my hour-long morning workout, I was building energy to store for later use; there was no way I was going to waste precious energy on *thinking* about cleaning my car from the earlier coffee mess when I could just *do it* when I left the gym. Energy is precious. Something as inconsequential as four or five ounces of spilled coffee was not worth expending double energy. I wasn't going to let a rotten 20 minutes spoil the remaining nineteen hours and forty minutes of my day.

Nothing in your life is going to change until you take action

Something in motion tends to stay in motion and something at rest tends to stay at rest unless acted upon by an outside force. Isaac Newton defined inertia as his first law in his *Philosophiæ Naturalis Principia Mathematica*, which states: The *vis insita*, or innate force of matter, is a power of resisting by which everybody, as much as in it lies, endeavors to preserve its present state, whether it be of rest or of moving uniformly forward in a straight line.

So basically, ain't nuthin' happenin' until you make it so! In order to get the life changing results you so deeply desire you must take action; and once you decide to take action the next natural question becomes, "how?" The answer, my friend, is just start. Once you're committed to the process the answers appear just as they're needed. I remember writing my first book back in 2003 – a friend of mine encouraged me through the whole process. Even then I had many starts and stops but not for reasons you may think. This was my very first book and I was clueless about the process. I actually stopped writing because I didn't know how I was going to get my book published. My friend advised me to keep writing; empty words of hope I thought. Why would I keep writing when this may end of being a waste of time? Boy, was I wrong. Once the book was completed I started talking it up within my network and before I knew it my book was on Amazon and being sold in Barnes and Noble stores across the country. People, places and situations appeared from the least likely places all in all to help my book. Once you make the effort and take the first step, I can promise you, what you need will appear and help you get from where you are to where you want to be.

This is a photo of me at the beginning of my journey; you can even see my tummy hanging down. I was so happy that I could balance on all fours. This is a beautiful memory. I've come so far. Imagine where I'd be now if I never started.

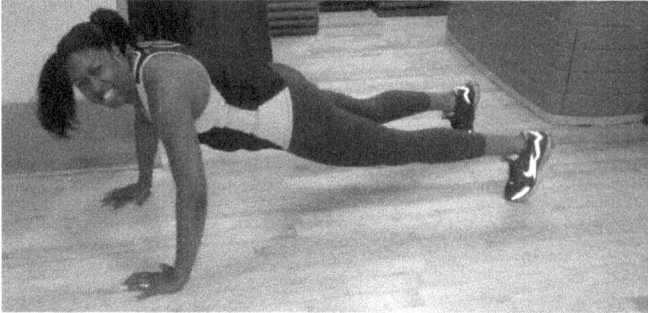

I can easily see my hands are not properly positioned, for a regular push up or a triceps push up, and my legs are wider than my shoulders; but at least I am on the floor trying. I remember when all I could do was lift my body a mere three inches off the floor; now I can drop and do pushups with ease. I may not be where I want to be, but I'm definitely not where I was. We all have to start somewhere, right?

Start slowly and quietly

Many newbies on the journey go in so amped up that they throw caution to the wind. Yes, I strongly encourage you to start working out as soon as you feel ready but realize you cannot run 5 miles on a treadmill when they last time you worked out was in high school. You'll hurt yourself and we definitely don't want that. This is not a game and you can do some serious damage to your body if you're not careful. Start slowly and quietly; slowly, so you don't hurt yourself and quietly so you're not judged. It's freeing when you take control of your life but it will become more difficult to do so under extra scrutiny. Remember, I started in the back of the class by the door. No one knew who I was and it wasn't until I became more comfortable at the gym did I start to spread my wings a bit.

Tips to Get Moving

1. Walk. It's something you can do anywhere and at any time. Even walk in the rain, you'll walk more quickly and burn more calories.

2. Stretch Up. Stand with both feet flat on the floor no wider than your shoulders and reach your arms up as high as they can go. Reach, reach, reach, reach, reach, reach. As you're looking up, and if you have good balance, lift your heels off of the floor and keep reaching. You should feel a good stretch in the back of your legs.

3. Stretch Right. Standing with both feet flat on the floor no wider than your shoulders, put your left hand on the left side of your waist, raise your right arm straight up towards the ceiling, tip from the hip towards the left side of your body, gently curve your right arm and lean towards your left. Reach, reach, reach, reach, reach as you're counting to ten; then slowly bring your arm back to the top, straighten it out, pull it down and rebalance yourself.

4. Stretch Left. Standing with both feet flat on the floor no wider than your shoulders, put your right hand on the right side of your waist, raise your left arm straight up towards the ceiling, tip from the hip towards the

right side of your body, gently curve your left arm and lean towards your right. Reach, reach, reach, reach, reach as you're counting to ten; then slowly bring your arm back to the top, straighten it out, pull it down and rebalance yourself.

5.  Push Ups. Remember your high school gym teacher telling the girls they could do girl-push-ups on their knees? The truth is push-ups are simple enough to be done at any fitness level and no matter what your gender is the ultimate goal is to be able to lift your body off of the floor using the strength in your arms. If you're unable to get on the floor start by leaning against the wall and pushing yourself away.

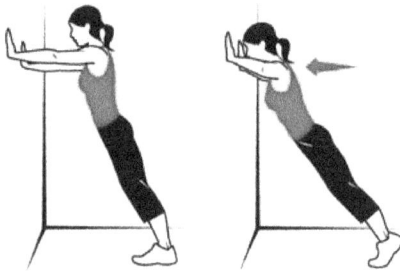

As you gain strength, move to the floor with bended knees.

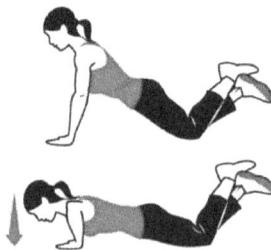

And finally, drop to the floor with your legs straight and push your body up.

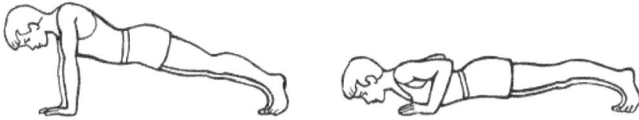

6. Lunges. There are three main leg muscle groups, the quadriceps (the muscle on the top/outer part of your thigh), the hamstring (the inner/back part of your thigh), and the calf (the muscle on the back of your leg below your knee). Lunges are great because not only do they work the three main leg muscle groups but they also work on your butt!

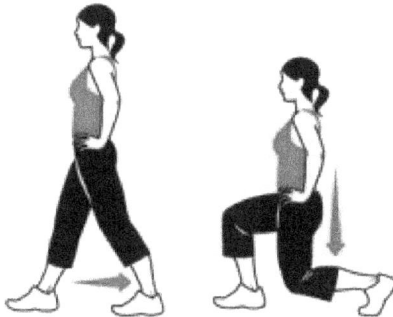

Stand straight up and use one leg to take a huge step back, slightly bending the hind leg. Bend both legs at the knees until they are both at 90 degree angles. If your front knee extends too far over your big tow then you have not stepped you hind leg back far enough. Keeping your weight in the heel of the planted foot, push your body back up slowly into the standing position you started in. Repeat on the other leg.

7. Hovers. A great way to get rid of belly fat is to strengthen the muscles underneath that fat. Your core and your "abs" are not the same thing; your abdominal area is only one part of your total core area. Our core is the home base for all of our bodily movement. If your core is not strong then your body will use, and possibly overuse, the lower back, knees and shoulders. This puts us at risk for other ailments; hovers, also known as planks are a great core strengthening exercise.

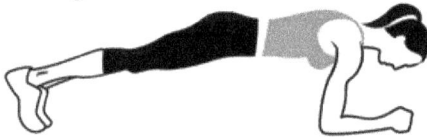

Lay on the floor totally flat with your arms stretched out in front of you like Superman; slide your elbows in towards your body keeping them close. When your elbows are at a 90 degree angle, climb up on your toes and lift your body up using the weight in your arms for stabilization. Stay there for 30 seconds intervals.

8. Standard Crunch. There are many, many variations of an abdominal crunch and I strongly recommend that you pay close attention to your body during this aspect of your workout because you can really hurt your neck and back if you're not careful. I started with a standard up-down crunch and then moved into a crunch with a twist. Lay on your back with your knees bent and your feet flat on the floor. You can either cross your arms across your chest or make your arms into wings by bending them so they are flat on the

floor and your middle finger is barely touching the inside of your ear. Push your lower back into the floor and roll your body up half way towards your knees then roll back down. Repeat. If you need to put a towel or a blanket under your lower back to reduce pressure, feel free to do so.

9.  Crunch with a twist. This type of abdominal workout builds additional strength on the sides of your core. Start off in the same position as a regular crunch – knees bent, feet flat on the floor, arms out like wings but instead of coming straight up, gently twist your body so that your shoulder reaches for the opposite knee. Repeat. If you need to put a towel or a blanket under your lower back, feel free to do so.

10. Squats. The more you strengthen your muscles the more calories you burn and squats are a great strength training exercise. Keep your feet should-width apart and your back straight with your arms by your side. As you lower your butt to the floor, raise your arms so they are directly in front of you while keeping your knees over your ankles as much as possible. Stay there for a few seconds, come on up into standing position and repeat. If your arms get tired that's okay; you're building up strength in your upper body too. I wasn't too keen on squats but once I noticed my butt getting more round and firm I became a squat addict…and you will too!

Don't let the initial aches and pains stop you from pressing on!

Stretching your body beyond what it's used to delivers an ample dose of aches and pains in the beginning. When I started taking classes on a stationary bike (also known as a Spin or cycling class) my tush hurt for a week and I could barely walk the first two days. I pressed on and now I take a one-hour class a few times a week and my tush doesn't hurt anymore. It took time for my body to adapt but it did, and yours will too.

Whitney Houston famously sang "Learning to love yourself is the greatest love of all." Self-love will get you through those tough moments after a grueling workout. No one else is better than you are, they may have started the journey before you but that doesn't make them better than you as a person. Serena Williams is a much better tennis player than I am because she started much sooner than me. Perhaps if I started as a child I could have been as great as she is. Serena is not a better person than me, she is better at what she does than me.

More often than not, we think and believe that others are better than us, when in reality they're not. It's all perception. We all have our insecurities and none of us is perfect. Everybody wants what everybody wants; better things, better features, better body parts or better whatever be happy with what you have. Use this time in your life to improve upon what God has given you to work with. You don't have to shout to the world you're on a diet; dig your heels in, do the work and let your body speak for itself.

# Chapter Five
# Get To Sleep

Slow down, sleep more is the blueprint of success
**Arianna Huffington, Founder and Editor-in-Chief
of the Huffington Post**

Sleep patterns are as personal as a finger print, so it's important you pay attention to your body to see how and under what conditions you sleep best, the most effectively and the most efficiently. When your body is at complete rest, your organs are not fighting against other activities to function. Sleep is known to restore the soul but it's also a time to rejuvenate your physical body. Sleep gives your body untethered permission to restore itself. You're actually honoring your body when you rest.

Lack of sleep produces more of the hormone ghrelin, which stimulates the feeling of hunger and less of the hormone leptin, which curbs the desire to eat, stable levels of each complement each other and balances the *desire* to eat with the actual *need* to eat. When you don't get enough sleep your leptin levels decrease which makes you want to eat more. When you're getting enough sleep, your leptin levels increase and decreases your desire to eat. Further, if you're comfortably sleeping six or more hours per night you likely won't rely on artificial snacks and caffeinated beverages to give you an energy jolt during low periods in your day.

## ⌐ Sleep restores the body

Our bodies are still working, even when we're nestled in a nice comfy bed with huge big blankets. If you've ever had a paper cut, after the initial sting, you probably washed your hands, put a band-aid on it, and kept life moving, right? Well, while you were busy living life your body was busy healing your cut, without any effort of your own; your body knew exactly what to do. Now, if you use your hands a lot during the day, like most people, you're likely compromising the speed of recovery of the paper cut because your hands are in and out of water, you're folding things, you're driving and other activities. When you're asleep, your body sends healing energy to the paper cut and everywhere else that needs repair. Physical health conditions may prevent a good night's sleep and if that's your experience then I strongly suggest you visit a physician. Sleep is spiritual, it connects you to your deeper self and if physical conditions are blocking the connection, professional help is required.

## ⌐ Sleep restores the soul

When we slumber, our soul often travels. Our bodies are complex but our soul is simple. Our soul is designed just as our bodies are, to restore itself. Our soul desires connection and to be connected to that which is right; but during our waking moments, our logic, thoughts and worldly desires prevents a stable connection between the essence of who we are (subconsciously) and what we actually want (consciously). While we are sleeping, our soul is reconnecting. Our soul is at work making things right so when we awaken we have all of the answers to successfully navigate life. If we cheat ourselves out of a good night's sleep we are really losing an opportunity to get ahead in life; on many levels.

Please turn off the television before you fall asleep at night. For years, I didn't allow my children to have a TV in their room; they hated it but this was non-negotiable. While our bodies are asleep it is in the most open state it can be – we are receptive to everything in our sleep especially if our soul is traveling. So, the dimension your mind is in and what its experiencing as you begin to drift plays a major role in how peaceful your rest is and the state you awaken in. If a horror movie, or even the news for that matter, is broadcasting as you're drifting to sleep that energy will infiltrate your aura and your body will absorb that energy. I guarantee your sleep will be broken, restless and not peaceful at all. If you fall asleep with the lights off you'll sleep much better; and if soft music is playing I can guarantee even a better night's sleep. Sleeping is a sacred experience and should be protected. Your sleep environment should also be protected; and if for some reason your sleep environment (which could be a bedroom, a living room, a den, a hallway or a jail cell) is less than ideal, protect it to the best of your ability until you can do better.

Personal issues may prevent you from having a good night's sleep; ironically, a good night's sleep is probably what you need to resolve challenging personal issues. Don't let looming bills or problems at work keep you awake at night. Go to sleep and allow your soul to do its work. That way when you awaken, you'll know what to do, when to do it and how to do it. The answer may not come the next morning but if you stay aware and alert, you'll know exactly how to handle every situation that comes your way. Everything that happens to us happens for our greatest good. Always.

🏃 Get better sleep the natural way

There are so many products on the market that promise a good night's sleep but I don't recommend any of them. Many have life-altering side effects and can further exacerbate challenges within your body. To avoid further complications, it is best to try sleeping techniques that don't involve pills or chemicals. The first thing you can do is to develop and practice a good sleep-time routine. I must shower or bathe before I go to bed at night or I will not be able to sleep well. Not because I'm a neat freak or anything but because a few years ago I went to sleep without taking a bath or shower and in the middle of the night I had a freak accident and broke my right arm. I didn't realize it was broken, I thought I was just in a lot of pain. A trip to the emergency room confirmed my suspicion and my arm was placed in a cast from my shoulder to my wrist. At that point, I couldn't take a comfortable shower whether I wanted to or not. I was so emotionally affected by that experience my mind won't settle in to rest unless I have showered or bathed before I turn it in for the night. I have literally convinced myself that I cannot experience a good night's sleep unless I am totally clean. Was that too personal? Anyway, a good bedtime routine can and will help you sleep better naturally. Even if your routine involves sex, a cup of tea, journaling or some other activity. Take time to figure out what you can do, naturally, to enjoy a better night's sleep.

In addition to massive benefits in other areas of your life, eating the right foods during the day can help you sleep better naturally. Avoid caffeine and sugar; they destroy the body and should technically be classified as drugs. I love a good cup of Starbucks now and then but I stopped drinking it for a while then one morning I enjoyed a cup - my heart didn't stop racing until almost 3-o'clock in the afternoon. I love coffee but now I only drink decaf; decaf is not totally caffeine free but it definitely contains much less than a regular cup of joe.

Prepare your body to rest well as night. If you want to sleep well at night then make sure you have a kick-ass day. Be fully engaged during the day, leave everything on the floor and give it all you've got; that way when it's time to take it down your body is really ready to rest. Eat nutrient rich foods during the day and make sure you have plenty of protein. Protein builds muscle and helps you feel fuller. When you're sleeping your body will use the stored protein to enhance the repairs it was going to make anyway. Not only does good daytime preparation include eating the right foods but exercising as well. To help your body relax at night engage your body to the max during the day, push past your limits and take your physical movement to the next level. You should be doing enough physical activity during the day that your body *wants* to crash at night. Let your body get exhausted enough to crave rest at nighttime. Simple exercises such as brisk walking or light yoga activities are enough to help you get better sleep at night if you're unable to blast your body physically during the day.

Some people have a reverse job schedule and work at night and need to sleep during the day; if this is you then you really need to make sure your physical exertion is pushed to the max. It's much more difficult to sleep during the daylight hours when everybody is at work. In these instances, you really have to retrain your body and this may take time. Again, I don't recommend any sleep aids but once you really understand your body you'll know exactly what to do to get good rest.

Develop your own personal sleeping plan. Above all else, know your body. If you're having problems sleeping at night, you probably already know what the problem is. Remember, your soul travels during your sleep time to plant in your spirit all of the answers you need in life. Your body is renewed daily so be patient and don't get too frustrated if you can't sleep well. Listen attentively and become one with yourself; over time you'll be fine and sleep much better.

# Chapter Six
## Your Zen Zone

You must find the pace inside of you where nothing is impossible.
**Deepka Chopra, Co-Founder The Chopra Center for Wellbeing**

Many of us are overstressed and pushed to our limits on a daily basis; and for the most part, there is little we can do to thwart the happenings that come our way. What we do have, however, is control over the manner in which we govern ourselves as we navigate through our journey. To successfully get through challenging situations in life it's critical to stay in the moment and be fully present. Meaning, don't overthink the situation and don't overanalyze every detail. Stay alert but not focused on every detail that chaos brings. The answers are right there. Every answer you'll need to come out victoriously on the other side rests within the details of the difficulty you're experiencing. The challenge is that many of us have not trained our minds to think that way; so to an untrained mind the situation seems to be a flood when it's really only a drip. It's during these heightened moments of anxiety that we may seek comfort in food and if not food then in other unhealthy and destructive things.

Zen is not a thing, it's a state of awareness and being. What it's not is something spooky or mystic or anti-Christian, actually, it's weightless living. The answers to change everything around you and shape the future lies within. **Zen occurs when you're weightless enough to access your inner power.**

Aromatherapy helps train the mind, yoga trains the body and meditation brings forth the power of your soul.

## Chapter Six / Part Two
## Aromatherapy

The colloquialism *music calms the savage beast* is often misquoted. Playwright William Congreve wrote in his 1697 tragedy *The Mourning Bride* "Music has charms to soothe a savage breast…" Music undeniably, alters moods, sets tones and shifts energy; there is none like it other than a soothing scent. The smell of something familiar or something warm can have just as much of an impact on human emotion and behavior as the sound of wind chimes blowing on a warm summer day.

Aromatherapy is the soothing inhalation of plant-derived essential oils to reduce stress, stabilize moods and relieve minor discomforts. When essential oils are applied topically, they're absorbed into our blood stream and can quickly soothe bruises and tender muscles as well as decrease inflammation. The global fragrance industry is estimated to rake in over $30-billion dollars per year and shows no sign of slowing down. The products net huge profits for manufacturers but for the consumer, it's a small price to pay for happiness. Smelling good makes you feel good and that's what everyone wants; they want to feel good, feel well and feel happy and aromatherapy is an affordable pleasure.

The use of essential oils can easily benefit your overall health and wellness, the key is finding a scent that works for you – a scent that takes you to that place. My husband knows just what to splash on to get things live and poppin' at my house! His natural scent infused under our favorite cologne definitely takes me there. You may have to experiment for a while to find a scent that works for you, have fun with it. Start with small bottles, and when you find the one that rocks best with your natural body fragrance go for it and buy a big bottle. I'm not a fan of florals like rose or gardenia, my preference is heavier scents like vanilla and sandalwood. Use what makes you happy. If you're a morning person you may want to use a different scent when you wake up than when you take it down for the night. The beauty of essential oils and aromatherapy in general is their unique ability to change how you feel. Your favorite scent will instantly grab you and make you happy. It's impossible to enjoy your favorite scent and be angry at the same time. It's impossible, trust me. Here are some common essential oils and their use.

## Allspice Berry

The oil has a warm, spicy-sweet aroma. It is used in spicy or masculine scents. It combines well with orange, ginger, patchouli and all of the spice oils including cinnamon, cassia and clove. Aromatherapy benefits: warming, cheering, comforting, nurturing.

## Amyris

Amyris is also known as West Indian sandalwood, although unrelated to the true Indian sandalwood. It has a woody, slightly sweet, balsamic aroma, suggestive of sandalwood. Amyris is used as a fragrance fixative-it slows the evaporation and dissipation of the fragrance it is added to. It blends well with cedar wood, jasmine and rose scents. Aromatherapy benefits: strengthening, centering.

## Anise

The oil of anise and star anise are often used and sold interchangeably because they are similar in aroma and chemical make-up. The primary constituent of both is anethole, a sweet substance that solidifies at room temperature. If this happens simply, warm the bottle in a warm water bath until the oil liquefies. Aromatherapy benefits: cheering, mildly euphoric.

## Basil

There are many types of basil: linalool basil, exotic basil and sweet basil. The odor of the linalool type is very green, floral-sweet and is most often used in expensive perfumes. The exotic type of basil is stronger with a hint of camphor. Sweet basil type combines both qualities in a floral-spicy aroma with a lasting herbal sweetness. Clary sage, bergamot and lime oil work well with basil oil. Aromatherapy benefits: clarifying, uplifting, energizing, refreshing.

## Bay

Bay oil is distilled from the leaves and small twigs of the bay rum tree. It has a powerful, spicy, sweet aroma with a distinctive clove note. It is used to produce bay rum fragrance and as a component of fresh, spicy scents. Aromatherapy benefits: clarifying, warming.

## Bergamot

Bergamot oil is cold-pressed from the peel of the nearly ripe fruit. The aroma of bergamot oil is fresh, lively, fruity and sweet. It is an excellent deodorizer. Aromatherapy benefits: uplifting, inspiring, confidence-building.

## Camphor

White is the grade preferred in scenting detergents, soaps, disinfectants, deodorants, room sprays and other domestic and household products. Aromatherapy benefits: clarifying, energizing, purifying.

## Cardamom Seed

The oil from a cardamom seed has a spicy, camphor-like aroma with floral undertones. It imparts a warm note to masculine scents and floral perfumes. It blends well with bergamot, frankincense, ylang-ylang, cedar wood and coriander. Aromatherapy benefits: warming, comforting, alluring.

## Carrot Seed

Carrot seed oil is distilled from the seed of the common carrot. Its aroma is dry-woody, somewhat sweet and earthy. In perfumery, carrot seed oil is appreciated for the interesting fatty-woody note it lends to oriental, fantasy, and nature-type perfumes. It is an excellent addition to skin care oils. Aromatherapy benefits: replenishing, nourishing, restoring.

## Cassia Bark

Cassia, or Chinese cinnamon, is the spice sold as cinnamon in the United States. Ceylon cinnamon is considered the true cinnamon in most of the world outside of the United States. The two are similar in taste, though Ceylon cinnamon has a sweeter, more delicate flavor. The oils of both contain cinnamic aldehyde as the major component, with cassia having the larger amount. Caution: Cassia oil is very irritating to the skin and should be handled with care. Aromatherapy benefits: comforting, energizing, warming.

## Cedar Wood

Red cedar wood essential oil actually comes from a type of juniper known as Juniperus virginiana, whose common name is eastern red cedar. The balsamic-woody aroma of cedar wood oil evokes a feeling of inner strength and centeredness. It is quite useful in times of emotional stress and anxiety to overcome feelings of powerlessness.

## Chamomile, German

The oil of German chamomile is also known as blue chamomile. The color of the oil is deep blue, turning green then brown with age and exposure to light. The odor is sweet, tobacco-like and fruity, apple-like. It adds a warm, long-lasting, rich undertone in perfumes. Chamomile is a mild, soothing oil and is popular in massage blends and other herbal preparations. Aromatherapy benefits: calming, relaxing, soothing.

## Chamomile, Roman

Roman chamomile contains only trace amounts of the intense blue component azulene, which gives German chamomile its color. This oil is commonly used in perfumery and blends well with bergamot, jasmine, neroli and clary sage, lending a warm, fresh note when added in small quantities. The aroma is not long-lasting like that of the German chamomile but it is a mild, soothing oil. Aromatherapy benefits: relaxing, calming.

## Chamomile, Wild

Wild or Moroccan chamomile is related to Roman chamomile. While the fragrance of these two are somewhat similar, wild chamomile is distinct enough to have earned its own place in perfumery. Wild chamomile has a fresh, herbal note and a rich, balsamic, sweet undertone which is very long-lasting. It blends well with woody fragrances like cypress, as well as citrus oils and musk scents like angelica. Aromatherapy benefits: soothing, nurturing.

## Cinnamon Bark

Also known as Ceylon cinnamon, this is the true cinnamon of world commerce. Its aroma is similar to cassia, or Chinese cinnamon. The aroma of Ceylon cinnamon is preferred to cassia for perfume where it gives a warm, floral-enhancing effect. Cinnamon oil blends well with oriental-woody notes and is often combined with frankincense. It is a skin irritant and should be handled with care. Aromatherapy benefits: comforting, warming.

## Cinnamon Leaf

Cinnamon leaf oil is distilled from the leaves of the same tree that produces cinnamon bark oil. The aroma is more reminiscent of cloves than cinnamon due to the large amount of eugenol in the oil. It is often used in Oriental fragrances. Use with care, cinnamon leaf can irritate the skin. Aromatherapy benefits: refreshing, vitalizing.

## Citronella

There are two types of citronella essential oil: the Java type and the Ceylon type. While the grass that produces the Java type oil is grown in many parts of the tropical world, the Ceylon type is cultivated in Sri Lanka. The oils produced from the two types of grasses vary somewhat in composition and aroma. The odor of Ceylon citronella is fresh, grassy and warm-woody. It is preferred for scenting outdoor sprays, room sprays and household products. Java oil has a sweeter, more floral aroma which is preferred in perfumery. Aromatherapy benefits: purifying, vitalizing.

## Clary Sage

Clary sage oil has a spicy, hay-like, bittersweet aroma. It combines well with coriander, cardamom, citrus oils, sandalwood, cedarwood, geranium and lavandin. The aroma of clary sage is long-lasting and the oil is valued as a fixative for other scents. Aromatherapy benefits: centering, euphoric, visualizing.

## Clove Bud

The best clove oil is distilled from the whole dried flower buds of the clove tree. Inferior oils are distilled from the leaves and stems and are sometimes sold as clove oil without any designation of the source. Clove bud oil has a powerful, spicy-fruity, warm, sweet aroma. Clove oil is highly irritating to the skin and should be handled with caution. Aromatherapy benefits: warming, comforting.

## Coriander Seed

Coriander oil has a delightful fragrance: spicy, aromatic, pleasantly sweet, not unlike bergamot orange. It blends well with clary sage, bergamot, cinnamon bark, jasmine and frankincense for use in spicy, masculine perfumes or light, floral colognes. Aromatherapy benefits: nurturing, supportive.

## Cypress

Cypress oil has a refreshing, spicy, juniper and pine needle-like aroma and is often used as a modifier in pine fragrances. It blends well with lavender, clary sage, citrus and Angelica. Aromatherapy benefits: purifying, balancing.

## Eucalyptus

Of the 300 species of eucalyptus trees in the world, Eucalyptus globulus is the best known. Eucalyptus has long been used in topical ointments such as liniments and salves. Aromatherapy benefits: purifying, invigorating.

## Frankincense

Various species of frankincense trees grow wild throughout Western India, Northeastern Africa and Southern Saudi Arabia. The oil is distilled from the gum resin that oozes from incisions made in the bark of the trees. The oil is spicy, balsamic, green-lemon-like and peppery. It modifies the sweetness of citrus oils such as orange and bergamot. It is also the base for incense type perfumes and is important in Oriental, floral, spice and masculine scents. Aromatherapy benefits: calming, visualizing, meditative.

## Geranium

This oil is one of the most important perfumery oils and is an important ingredient in all types of fragrances. It has a powerful, leafy-rose aroma with fruity, mint undertones. Bourbon oil, from the island of Reunion, is considered the finest grade, and has the best staying power. It is used in skin care products for both its fragrance and its toning, cleansing properties. Aromatherapy benefits: soothing, mood-lifting, balancing.

## Ginger
Ginger oil has a warm, spicy-woody odor. It blends well with spice and citrus oils. Aromatherapy benefits: warming, strengthening, anchoring.

## Grapefruit
Grapefruit oil is often cold-pressed from the peel of the common grapefruit. It has a fresh, sweet, bitter, citrus aroma. It is used to scent citrus perfumes and colognes, soaps, creams and lotions. Aromatherapy benefits: refreshing, cheering.

## Jasmine
The fragrance of jasmine is a component in so many perfumes that there is an old saying: "No perfume is complete without jasmine." Artificial jasmine cannot begin to compete with the full, rich, honey-like sweetness of true jasmine, despite the efforts of the best perfume chemists in the world. Great expense goes into producing pure jasmine oil. The flowers must be hand-picked before dawn when the essence is at its peak, and large quantities are needed to produce small amounts of oil. Aromatherapy benefits: calming, relaxing, sensual, romantic.

## Juniper Berry
Juniper berry oil is distilled from the dried ripe berry of the juniper tree. Juniper berry oil has a fresh, warm, balsamic, woody-pine needle odor. It is used with citrus oils in room sprays and in masculine and outdoorsy perfumes, after shaves and colognes. Aromatherapy benefits: supportive, restoring.

## Lavender

Lavender oil is used in baths, room sprays, toilet waters, perfumes, colognes, massage oils, sachets, salves, lotions and oils. It has a sweet, balsamic, floral aroma which combines well with many oils including citrus, clove, patchouli, rosemary, clary sage and pine. Aromatherapy benefits: balancing, soothing, normalizing, calming, relaxing, healing.

## Lemon

Cold-pressed lemon oil is a much better oil than distilled. The scent is evocative of the fresh ripe peel. Lemon oil in the bath or in massage oils should be well diluted as it can cause skin irritation. Caution: avoid using the oil in body care products when going out into the sun as it can cause redness and burning of the skin. Aromatherapy benefits: uplifting, refreshing, cheering.

## Lemon Eucalyptus

The aroma of Eucalyptus citriodora is similar to the aroma of citronella. Both contain citronellal as a major component. Eucalyptus citriodora has a fresh, rosy, grass-like aroma. It blends well with eucalyptus globulus, moderating that oils somewhat medicinal aroma. Aromatherapy benefits: purifying, invigorating.

## Lemongrass

Lemongrass oil is distilled from a tropical grass native to Asia. It has a powerful, lemony, grassy aroma. It is used in insect repellents, room sprays, soaps and detergents. Aromatherapy benefits: vitalizing, cleansing.

## Lime

Two types of lime oil are commonly sold; distilled and cold-pressed. Distilled oil is pale yellow or clear in color with a perfumey-fruity, limeade aroma. Pressed oil, is yellowish to green in color, with a rich, fresh, lime peel aroma. While pressed lime oil is produced in smaller quantities and is more expensive than distilled lime oil, it is preferred in aromatherapy. Aromatherapy benefits: refreshing, cheering.

## Marjoram, Sweet

Sweet marjoram is distilled from the leaves and flowering tops of the same plant that produces the culinary herb. The aroma of the oil is warm and spicy, with a hint of nutmeg. It is used in masculine and herbal-spicy perfumes and colognes. Aromatherapy benefits: warming, balancing.

## Myrrh

Natural myrrh resin is one of the oldest known perfumery materials. The oil has a balsamic, warm and spicy aroma that blends well in Oriental, woody and forest-type perfumes. It is also used in ointments and other skin care products. Myrrh was used as incense and in embalming preparation in ancient Egypt. Aromatherapy benefits: centering, visualizing, meditative.

## Neroli

Oil of neroli is distilled from the flowers of the bitter orange tree. It has a very strong, refreshing, spicy, floral aroma and is one of the most widely used flower oils in perfumery. It is an ingredient in eau de cologne and blends well with citrus oils and floral oils. Neroli is also used in premium natural cosmetic preparations such as massage oils, skin creams and bath oils. Aromatherapy benefits: calming, soothing, sensual.

## Nutmeg

Nutmeg oil is distilled from whole, dried nutmegs that have been cut into small particles and pressed to remove the fixed oil, also known as nutmeg butter. The oil has the characteristic aromatic, volatile, oily-spicy fragrance of whole nutmegs. Nutmeg oil is a component in men's fragrances and spicy perfumes. Aromatherapy benefits: rejuvenating, uplifting, energizing.

## Orange, Sweet

More sweet orange oil is produced than any other citrus oil. Two kinds of sweet orange oil are available: distilled or expressed. Distilled oil is a byproduct of juice making and has an inferior aroma. It is often used as an adulterant in expressed or pressed oil. It has a lively, fruity, sweet aroma. It is used to scent fruity and eau de cologne fragrances. All citrus oils are quick to deteriorate and should be stored in a cool, dry, dark area in full containers. Aromatherapy benefits: cheering, refreshing, uplifting.

## Patchouli

Used in countless perfumes and fragrances, patchouli is noted for its long-lasting fragrance and fixative ability. It borders on the exotic and even the name patchouli evokes images of heady aromas, dark, rich colors, candlelight, incense and intrigue. The aroma is very intense; it can be described as earthy, rich, sweet, balsamic, woody and spicy. Patchouli oil is one of the few essential oils that improve with age. Aromatherapy benefits: romantic, soothing, sensual.

## Peppermint

Peppermint has a powerful, sweet, menthol aroma which, when inhaled undiluted, can make the eyes water and the sinuses tingle. Aromatherapy benefits: vitalizing, refreshing, cooling.

## Pine

Pine oil is distilled from the twigs and needles of the Scotch pine that grows throughout much of Europe and Asia. It has a fresh, resinous, pine needle aroma. The oil is used to scent a number of household and personal care products such as room sprays, detergents, vaporizer liquids, cough and cold preparations and masculine perfumes. When used in skin care preparations, pine oil should always be well diluted as it can be irritating to sensitive skin. Aromatherapy benefits: refreshing, invigorating.

## Rose

Rose oil is one of the oldest and best known of all the essential oils. The fragrance of rose is associated with love. It is warm, intense, immensely rich and rosy. It is used in perfumes to lend beauty and depth. A drop or two in a massage, facial or bath oil is luxurious and soothing. The oil is used in skin creams, powders and lotions. Aromatherapy benefits: romantic, supportive, gently uplifting.

## Rosemary

Rosemary is known as the herb of remembrance. The plant produces an almost colorless essential oil with a strong, fresh, camphor aroma. It's used in many citrus colognes, forest and Oriental perfumes, and eau de cologne. Rinses for dark hair often contain rosemary, as do room deodorants, household sprays, disinfectants and soaps. Aromatherapy benefits: clarifying, invigorating.

## Rosewood

Rosewood, or bois de rose, is a tropical tree growing wild in the Amazon basin. It has a sweet-woody, floral-nutmeg aroma that finds extensive use in fantasy-type perfumes and colognes. It is also used to scent soaps, creams, lotions, bath oils and massage oils. Aromatherapy benefits: gently strengthening, calming.

## Sandalwood

Sandalwood oil has a sweet-woody, warm, balsamic aroma that improves with age. The essential oil blends wonderfully with most oils, especially rose, lavender, neroli and bergamot. Sandalwood oil is also an excellent cleansing, astringent addition to massage and facial oils, bath oils, aftershaves, lotions and creams. Aromatherapy benefits: relaxing, centering, sensual.

## Spearmint

Aromatherapists use spearmint to energize the mind and body. A few drops in bath water has a refreshing effect while a facial steam of spearmint oil helps cleanse and tighten pores. Aromtherapy benefits: refreshing, cooling, vitalizing.

## Spruce

Several species of evergreen conifer trees are used to produce this pleasant, balsamic, sweet, evergreen-scented essential oil. The oil is used as a fragrance for household products by itself or with other pine needle oils to produce a fresh pine scent. Applications include air fresheners, room sprays, disinfectants, detergents and soaps. It blends well with cedarwood, galbanum, rosemary and all pine needle oils. Aromatherapy benefits: clarifying, vitalizing.

## Tangerine

Tangerine oil is pressed from the peel of ripe fruit. It is an orange-colored oil with the vibrant fragrance of fresh tangerines. The oil is used in colognes and occasionally in perfumes. (See Mandarin Orange.) Aromatherapy benefits: cheering, uplifting.

## Tea Tree

The leaf of the tea, or ti tree had a long history of use by the indigenous peoples of Australia before tea tree was discovered by the crew of the famous English explorer James Cook. The aroma of the oil is warm, spicy, medicinal and volatile. It is occasionally used to scent spicy colognes and aftershaves. It blends well with lavandin, rosemary and nutmeg oils. Aromatherapy benefits: cleansing, purifying, uplifting.

## Thyme, White

White thyme starts out as red thyme oil that has been further refined and redistilled to remove the constituents that produce the red color. The aroma and action of white thyme oil are a bit milder than that of red thyme. Both are used to scent soaps, colognes and aftershaves. Caution: Thyme oil can be irritating to the skin and should be used cautiously. Aromatherapy benefits: cleansing, purifying, energizing.

## Vanilla

This is one of my favorite scents. The lingering aroma is slightly heavy, woodsy and mixes well with wood-type scents. Aromatherapy benefits: calming, comforting.

## Vetiver

The aroma is rich, woody, earthy and sweet. It improves with age. Vetiver oil is used extensively in perfumery for its fixative effects as well as its fragrance. Aromatherapy benefits: supportive, grounding.

## Wintergreen

This oil was once an important perfumery and flavoring material, but has been replaced by less expensive and more reliable supplies of synthetic methyl salicylate. It is used in toothpaste and mouthwash Aromatherapy benefits: refreshing, bracing, invigorating.

## Ylang Ylang Extra

Ylang ylang oil is distilled from the early morning, fresh-picked flowers of the cananga tree. The distillation process is interrupted at various points and the oil accumulates is removed. The first oil to be drawn off is the highest quality and is graded "extra." Ylang ylang extra has an intense floral, sweet, jasmine-like, almost narcotic aroma. Aromatherapy benefits: sensual, euphoric.

There are hundreds of essential oils available in the marketplace with many different uses; some shouldn't be used on infants while others should not be ingested. Make sure you review all of the precautions before ingesting or topically applying an essential oil, whether directly or indirectly via lotion or a cream. Have fun with them! Sample as many as you can to see which scent resonates with your soul the most.

## Chapter Six / Part Three
## Yoga

Considered by many as an exercise fad or something religious, yoga practice has in fact helped thousands of people improve their physical and mental fitness. The practice of yoga has been around for more than four thousand years and its origins can be traced back to India where even today, it is considered as a highly valued practice to reach a state of enlightenment. A five-minute yoga exercise can perk you up and recharge your body with the energy you lost for the whole day. You relax and at the same time you stretch!

After Hurricane Sandy smashed the east coast in 2012, I relocated my part-time wellness practice from Hoboken, New Jersey into a four-story mixed-use brownstone in Harlem. The top floor housed the private residence of the owner, the second floor featured an amazing yoga studio and open space office and the first floor provided event space adjacent to the dining room and a kitchen. I offered the space to a pastor who was seeking a location to shoot her new television show; she toured the space and loved it. We invited her guests to the shoot, many of whom were pastors themselves and as they arrived, I offered them herbal tea made by the owner of the house and offered them a tour. As soon as they realized they were in a yoga studio the energy of the entire place changed. I physically saw the energy change – it was something I had never seen before and it was difficult for me to identify with at the time. They gracefully declined a tour; I thought they just wanted to get down to business and move on with the shoot. A few days later my friend, the pastor, told me they chastised her for using a yoga studio to shoot her Christian television show. I thought she was joking. How could anybody who knows anything about yoga think yoga and meditation is anything other than reconnecting with yourself and your highest energy. Yoga is not about praying to an elephant, a goose or standing on one leg and chanting to witches. She told me one of her pastor friends told her that people that practice yoga meditate, chant and say things while they are praying. My response was, "And don't they speak in tongues?" I wasn't trying to be disrespectful but I mean really. Humans have a tendency to condemn that which is unknown or unfamiliar to them. This section of my book hopes to demystify the practice of yoga and share with you how it can greatly benefit your overall health and wellbeing. Don't be scared, yoga can and will help you mentally and physically. Open up and allow yourself to experience new and exciting things. Let your body tingle with excitement a little.

Across the globe, the popularity of yoga is due to its many health benefits along with its associated use with asanas (postures) of Hatha Yoga as fitness exercises. Besides reaching a spiritual state of enlightenment, yoga can also help you reach a better understanding of not only your body but of your inner-self as well.

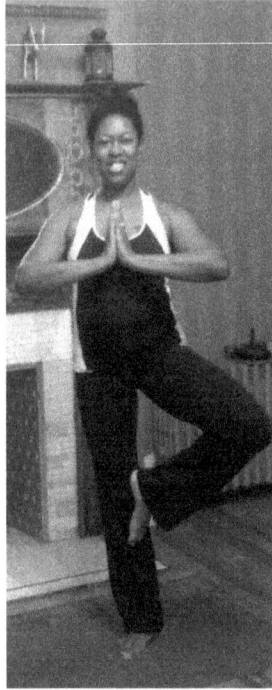

*Here I am learning tree pose. This move helps to strengthen my legs and better balance; metaphysically, this pose helps with balance in other areas of my life too. My left leg should be higher up my inner right thigh but, hey, I was just learning. Now I can rock this pose.*

When practicing yoga, you'll concentrate on body positioning, breathing and meditation; proper body positioning and movement controls the energy flow within your body, breathing controls your inflow and outflow of energy and meditation grounds your energy. Besides getting that ideal toned figure you've dreamed of, yoga will help you look and feel taller, good posture is so important.

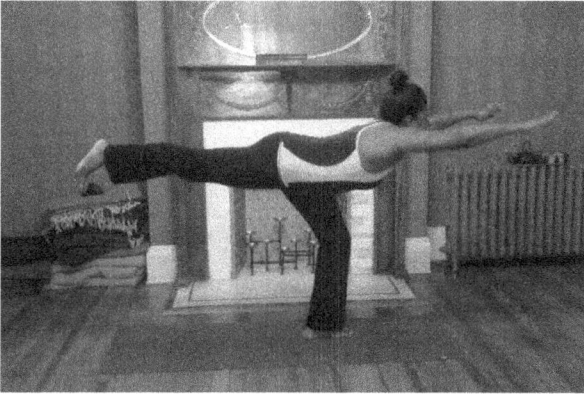

*Here I am learning Warrior III. Warrior III is a great post to help strengthen the abdomen, legs and butt.*

Yoga is a transformative art, and deceptively simple. It integrates your breath and consciousness with physical stretches, that when in a relaxed state increases in intensity. As you inhale your body takes in energy; as you exhale into a pose the stored energy provides a gentle enough force to help you sink into and more importantly stay in your pose. In yoga, through the breath, and focusing on it within our body, we come to a greater understanding of both our body and ourselves. We begin a more conscious relationship with our individuality. We meet that unique expression of ourselves that manifests at that precise moment. At that point, we're able to begin a process of changing that which is blocking the vital flow of our energy and holding our success hostage. Yoga is a journey of discovery, one that's not based on external idealism; even if that idea is represented in that moment by the yoga posture we are trying to do. Don't strain to get into a posture, be gentle with your mind and your body and the posture will come. Consider the posture the outcome and the practice of yoga as the journey.

The asanas are a way of preparing ourselves to more fully meet the challenges of life in a way that does not throw us off balance, and increases our capacity to adapt to those changes that are inherent in life. They allow us to be more sensitive and aware to what is really going on inside us, and in life itself. This growing self-knowledge then provides us with a more complete picture in which our responses to whatever situations confront us more accurately reflects what is truly present. This deeper engagement that goes far beyond the emptiness of pop-culture gives is power. When we are distracted or preoccupied with doubts, worries, and fears, and even hope that is attached to an outcome, the vital energy of our whole being is leaking and becomes diffused. Through yoga we're able to see our power and tap into at-the-ready no matter what is going on around us. Yoga is the energetic foundation of self-mastery.

### How to start your yoga practice

Yoga instructors are highly trained fitness professionals, so this is one program I do not recommend you begin at home or alone. Regardless if you choose to take a class at your local gym or community center, make sure the instructor is certified. If there aren't any studios or gyms in your area that offer classes, consider hiring a private instructor or getting some DVD's; you can even stream yoga classes online if that works for you. The key is starting. Many of the poses were quirky and I was very clumsy in the beginning but I am so much better now and I am so grateful I had the courage to start!

## What to wear for yoga

Since you'll be doing a lot of stretching I recommend clothing that stays in place. Flowy tops and loose fitting bottoms can get you tangled up as you move into poses. I don't recommend a regular bra – a sports bra with no metal finishes will work best. Tiny metal attachments may pinch your skin as you twist. I also recommend good underwear that won't chafe and moves with you. Yoga is typically practiced in bare feet so you don't have to worry about sneakers but you may want to purchase yoga socks. These little dandies have rubber bottoms and are a nifty way to keep you from slipping as you move in and out of poses. Sometimes I even wear yoga inspired t-shirts that feature empowering sayings; these t-shirts and tank tops remind me to feel good about myself and the changes occurring in my mind and body.

## The best yoga accessories

Your yoga mat will provide a center stage for all exercises and will serve as a focal point during all meditations and routines. I actually use two mats so I am protected from floor in vertical and horizontal seated positions. Buy one that has some thickness to it. Some inexpensive mats are paper thin and not very comfortable once they're in use. Your yoga mat is your grounding source during meditation, make sure it's comfortable.

Other yoga accessories include wool blankets that can be rolled and placed on the floor or under your back during deep breathing exercises. Some yoga students use blocks to assist with poses if their muscles aren't limber enough to reach maximum position. Colorful, long rubber straps are used to help maintain a pose for a longer period than if no strap is used. Sandbags can be used during class to accelerate muscle development. I've never used sandbags during a class but I know some advanced yoga students who have. Aside from the physical benefits of yoga, its quiet and deep relaxation techniques will help you maintain a more calm demeanor and better state of mind in all areas of your life especially in stressful situations. Stress kills and I want you to live a happy and long life.

## Chapter Six / Part Four
## Meditation

Sometimes we all feel like we're unable get a clear thought out, and that's because we cant! Between work, kids, Facebook, Instagram, Twitter, LinkedIn, the dog and grandma our brains are too cluttered and there's no room left for thoughts to flow freely. We can't possibly process another thought because there's simply not enough space. Even dirty dishes are vying for our attention. It's damn near impossible to fully think anything though nowadays. I once heard the difference between rich people and poor people is not about their respective net worth; it's that rich people have time to think. Remember when I shared how I quit my job in the beginning of this book, I knew then, if I kept going at that pace I was going to explode. Although I didn't have as much money as I would have liked once I quit my job; what I did have was time to think and plan and grow. Having money for the sake of having money is meaningless, having money to give you time to enjoy life and think and ponder gives money its true value.

Meditation and the art of meditating gives you a wonderful opportunity to release all that binds and welcome all that heals. I thought meditation was corny and only for real religious people until I hit a wall and my therapist suggested it. She told me that I was crashing and burning because I overthought everything and my brain and my body weren't designed for the way I was using them. I hoped for some prescribed miracle pill to make me feel better and all I received was her prescription for yoga and meditation. I gave meditation a shot and I'm a much better person because of it.

When I first sat down to meditate, I felt silly and goofy. I didn't know if I was supposed to be sitting against a wall, on the floor in a chair or what. Was I supposed to be chanting something, taking short breaths, long breaths or a mix of the two? I didn't know what the hell I was doing. So I went online and looked up how to start meditating. It was fascinating. There are some real meditation enthusiasts out there, all sharing tips from their perspective. Now you can add me to that list because I swear by meditating a few times a week.

When I got started I focused on three areas; my position, my breath and my thoughts.

**Positioning.** I sat flat on the floor with my back against the wall and my legs stretched out in front of me. This was slightly uncomfortable but this is the position I was led to. You may be led to sit, or stand, in some other position; do what feels right to you.

**Breathing.** I slowly inhaled through my nose and slowly exhaled through my mouth. I took the deepest breaths I could. This was challenging because it forced me to slow everything down. I didn't realize how constantly revved up I was until I tried to consciously slow my breathing down.

**Thoughts.** The more I focused on my breathing, the more thoughts flooded my mind. I began thinking about stuff that had no bearing on anything in my life at that time. This was very telling; it was during my first attempt at meditating that I realized how cluttered my life and my mind were.

My only focus during that first session was the blackness of the inside of my eyelids. I stayed there and refused to move. It was very difficult because I wanted to jump up at every ding of my cell phone and jot down notes of random thoughts in my head, but I didn't. It took almost 15 minutes to get calm. As I stood, I felt a little dizzy but I was determined to give it another go. Start small, maybe 2-3 minutes each time; as your meditation practice improves you'll be able to meditate for longer periods of time. If you can even get in ten minutes a day, you'll see a noticeable difference in your life because of the way you handle certain situations. People who meditate find it easier to give up negative habits and focus on the here and now. Over time you'll notice that irritable nuances don't bother you anymore. Keep your mind and your life as clutter free as possible; and if you don't have time to meditate activate your favorite essential oil to refocus on the happiness in your life. Namaste!

# Chapter Seven
## Eating Well on a Tight Budget

The most remarkable thing about my mother is that for
30 years she served the family nothing but leftovers.
The original meal has never been found.
**Calvin Trillin, Food Writer and Journalist**

For many, a limited food budget can be perceived as a major roadblock to healthy eating; I believe the roadblock is more about access to healthy foods than finances because we have a choice of what we buy when we shop. Unfortunately, the prevalence of low priced fast foods makes eating unhealthy foods quick, convenient and easy. It's cheaper for my husband and I to eat dinner at a casual dining restaurant during happy hour than to go home and cook; even though that's not the healthiest dinner option. The key to eating well on a tight budget is healthy foods education and planning. Here are a few tips to help you in those areas:

**Replace meat with beans and other protein alternatives.** Eating less meat and more beans and lentils is a good way to save money on your food budget while still getting the protein you and your family need. Try experimenting with vegetarian recipes for interesting ways to use these non-meat alternatives.

**Resist the affects of food marketing and advertising.** Sadly, the most marketed consumable products are the least healthy. When was the last time you saw an ad for apples? Food and beverage companies spend billions of dollars marketing unhealthy, high-profit foods to kids and adults. I believe this type of predatory marketing should be illegal, but it's not. Buy what you know is healthy not what the advertisers says is right. The term *healthy* is very subjective and is left to wide interpretation because the federal government hasn't set an industry-wide or national standard; hopefully a standard that's beneficial to consumers is forthcoming.

**Grow your own food.** Did you know some local cities have zoned community gardens illegal? Yup, I know, that's crazy right. Do you want to you why? Because food manufacturers are engaging in dubious deals with legislators. Why should it be illegal for communities to grow their own food? Well, I can come up with several reasons, here are two; 1) the more people become educated about food and nutrition the healthier they'll eat and food manufacturers will make less money; 2) the more people grow their own food the less likely they'll depend on food manufacturers and food manufacturers will earn less money. I hope you see this is all about money. They want us to eat unhealthy and they want us to eat poorly because it keeps the economy going. Even growing your own spices is a start; we grow basil and other herbs right in our kitchen. A simple herb garden can easily grow in a windowsill or similar small space. There are kits available for just a few dollars that contain the seeds, pots and other items needed to start; or you can save even more money by buying the seeds and planters yourself. Cooking with herbs and spices is a great way to enjoy healthy eating on a budget. Spices and herbs flavor dishes without the need for heavy sauces, butter or other high fat preparations. Growing your own herbs greatly decreases the ingestion of toxins and pesticides that are ever-present in so many foods purchased at the grocery store.

**Buy the healthiest food you can afford.** Just about everyone wants to eat better, and in a perfect world money wouldn't be an issue but sadly it is. It is important, however, to buy the healthiest food you can afford, whether you are cooking for yourself or for a growing family.

**Buy what's in season and locally grown.** Another excellent way to save money while still eating a healthy diet is to buy fresh fruits and vegetables when they are in season in your local area. Buying locally grown produce is often the best way to guarantee freshness and quality, and in-season produce is generally less expensive since it does not need to be shipped hundreds or even thousands of miles.

**Healthy doesn't necessarily mean organic.** Most fruits, vegetables and beans are low cost and have a high nutritional value. Combining these two important features is a great way to make your budget stretch while providing your body with the nutrition it craves and needs. Many foods are labeled *organic* and aren't; so in all actuality, you just may be spending more money on regular products. Yes, another marketing gimmick created by food manufacturers. In order for a food to be labeled *USDA (United States Department of*

*Agriculture) Certified Organic,* it must pass the standards of the National Organic Standards Board, which consists of members of the organic community appointed to advise the USDA on regulatory topics.[1] [1]Source USDA.gov

**Mix exotic foods with staples to create new meals.** To make a healthy meal more appealing buy a variety of exotic fruits and other food items you've never tried before and mix them with your shopping staples to create a colorful and eclectic new meal. Why not make your next trip to the grocery store an adventure? Use grocery store sales to stock up on staples like whole grain cereals, breads and whole wheat flour to combine with your new food finds. In addition to in-store sales and manufacturers coupons, many grocery store chains offer customer loyalty cards which allow customers to save money on products they buy regularly. Since most of these programs are free, there is really no downside to their use.

**Cook meals at home and limit eating out.** Everyone wants to eat healthier, but there are so many temptations in today's fast-food, drive-through world; healthy eating can be very difficult and expensive if meals are not planned. The key is making healthy meals as easy to eat as unhealthy ones. To kick-start my fitness journey, I gave up all sugar for five days and giving up sugar meant more than just the sweetened condensed milk I use in my coffee every morning or the occasional chocolate chip cookie in the afternoon; it also meant the sugar that was contained in poultry seasoning and other secret hiding places. Many packaged foods contain an overabundance of ingredients that appeal to our taste buds and not necessarily what is best for our heart and overall health. I cook at home as much as I can because I want to know what I am eating, how the food is prepared and how it will affect my body. Food is intimate and personal; your body-temple inside and out.

**Cook in volume.** Cooking in large quantities, even if your family is small is a great way to save time and money. Cooking large pots of stews, soups, pasta dishes, chili and casseroles can be a huge time saver because you can freeze the leftovers for meals later in the week or even the week after next. When freezing leftovers, however, it is important to label the containers carefully, using freezer tape and a permanent marker. Try to keep the oldest foods near the top to avoid having to throw away expired items.

**Use a crock-pot.** Convenience devices are a huge time saver for busy families. Many delicious and healthy recipes can be started in the morning and left to cook all day in a crock-pot or slow cooker. In addition to crock-pot fare, spend time making extra meals on the weekends and store them in single serve microwave safe containers; to allow everyone to eat portion-controlled meals on their own schedule.

**Modify what you're already going eat.** Healthier eating doesn't have to mean making a radical change. There are very simple things you can do, such as cutting the skin from your chicken breast or trimming the fat from your favorite steak to significantly reduced your fat intake. Small incremental and consistent changes equals big, big results.

**Eat smaller meals and portions.** Train your body to eat smaller portions so you can still feel full and satisfied at the end of your meal. Your meal-time goal should be, eat-to-live and not live-to-eat. My body has now adapted to smaller meals and I'm rarely hungry. It's mind over matter; remember, you're in total control of what you put in your mouth.

**Stretch your meals.** It's possible to cook and use a little creativity to make one meal last for two or more meals. Why not make expensive skirt steak go further by interspersing chunks of less expensive beef tossed with slices of onions and red and green peppers.  Not only will you get twice as much food for your money, but you will enjoy a healthier meal as well.

**Brown bag your lunch.** When creating healthy brown bag lunches for yourself and your family, choose at least three choices from the following list.

> ➢ At least one fruit or vegetable - choose fresh, canned or frozen.  Some good choices are apples, bananas and oranges and fruit salad.

> ➢ A whole grain product - like bread, a tortilla shell, a bagel, pasta, rice or muffins.

> ➢ Milk or dairy products - like low fat or nonfat yogurt, skim milk, cheese or a yogurt drink or shake.

> ➢ Some type of protein - meat, fish, poultry, eggs, peanut butter, legumes or hummus

No matter what strategies you choose to make your food budget stretch when cooking healthy meals, I know you'll uncover the secrets to some delicious new recipes.

# Chapter Eight
## Your Trip To The Grocery Store

It's in your moments of decision that your destiny is shaped.
**Tony Robbins, Motivational Speaker**

Every healthy eating plan and weight loss strategy begins with a plan, and once that plan is crafted the decision is yours on how to proceed. Of course you must increase your physical exertion but part two of that, as we've been discussing throughout this book, is eating better. Learning to make smart choices when planning your meals is the key to the success of any healthy eating plan. **Your trip to the grocery store is sacred, this is where the magic happens.**

Before you even head out with your coupons and deals, start at home with a weekly food map. Planning meals well ahead of time allows you to take advantage of what is already in your freezer and helps to plan purchases around store sales and specials. A food map provides a sense of direction on what to buy, the quantities of what you're buying, what ingredients are needed for each meal and keeps you on track with your healthy eating plan and budget. Learn to be a smart shopper and purchase only what you need to help you on your journey, at least until you hit your goal weight. Remember, food manufacturers want you to shop recklessly, I'm here to help you be a super-smart shopper so you can lose weight and feel great!

🍴 Eat 75% for health and nutrition and 25% for taste

The diagram that follows is my actual food map. This is how I plan weekly meals for my husband and I; our children are grown so they don't really factor into what I buy for the house each week.

| DAY | 7am | 11am | 1pm | 3pm | 5pm | 7pm |
|-----|-----------|-------|-------|-------|--------|-------|
| 1 | Breakfast | Snack | Lunch | Snack | Dinner | Snack |
| 2 | Breakfast | Snack | Lunch | Snack | Dinner | Snack |
| 3 | Breakfast | Snack | Lunch | Snack | Dinner | Snack |
| 4 | Breakfast | Snack | Lunch | Snack | Dinner | Snack |
| 5 | Breakfast | Snack | Lunch | Snack | Dinner | Snack |
| 6 | Breakfast | Snack | Lunch | Snack | Dinner | Snack |
| 7 | Breakfast | Snack | Lunch | Snack | Dinner | Snack |

As you can see I plan everything – this is how I hit my goal weight, believe me. Now, understand that my breakfast may not be the same as my husband's breakfast and my dinner was a much smaller portion of his dinner but preparing my food map helped me get in and out of the grocery store with exactly what I needed and within my budget.

If you live alone than creating a food map should be pretty simple. If your meal plan suggests oatmeal and eggs for breakfast then you can buy one container of oatmeal and one dozen eggs and your breakfast is really set for the entire week. However, if you're a married mom of three then your breakfast column will look much differently. It may still contain oatmeal but since everyone else in your family may not be trying to lose weight you may also have to purchase bacon, sausage, ready-to-eat cereal, a gallon or two of milk and maybe even low-sugar breakfast bars for the kids to take on the school bus. It is a good idea to involve the entire family in creating the week's meal plan, get everyone's input and note everyone's favorite foods. This doesn't mean pizza every night and ice cream for dinner, it's still about healthy meals, but involving others in healthy meal planning is a great way to pique others' interest and help them understand why healthy eating is so important to you. It's also a good idea to get the entire family involved in the preparation of the meals. Even children too young to cook can help out by setting out the dishes, chopping vegetables, clearing the table and washing the dishes.

The beauty of meal mapping is its scalability. At the end of the day everyone should be eating three solid meals and two snacks per day. Again, the above diagram is the exact map I followed, complete with times I needed to eat. This worked miraculously for me. It helped me stay on track, eat when I was supposed to and not lose focus.

**Make a shopping list.** Anyone who has visited a supermarket lately knows how dangerous it is to enter the store without a shopping list in hand. Shopping without a sense of what you need and don't need opens you up to all manners of temptation, and most of those tempting foods are not nutritious. Additionally, those extra items can easily blow your food budget and leave you without the money to buy what you really need. A good trick is to keep a note pad near the table or refrigerator. Having the notepad within reach makes it easy to keep track of the foods you need the most.

Go through all of those flyers left at your doorstep. I live in an urban city and each week, on my porch is a plastic bag filled with coupons and deals from all of the local markets and some small businesses. Some of the same inserts can be found in the center of your local newspaper as well. Keeping track of these sales, and taking advantage of low prices is a great way to stock up on basics like pasta, rice, spaghetti sauce and other items that won't spoil. Keeping a good supply of staples on hand will avoid unnecessary trips to the store and also avoid the need to buy such items when they are not on sale. Once your pantry is full you can now spend a little extra on fresh fruits, vegetables and other healthy food items. In addition, locally grown, in-season fruits and vegetables are sometimes more of a bargain than out of season fruits and vegetables that are transported to your area.

Use coupons, but wisely. Manufacturer's coupons can lead to great deals when used on products you already buy; and when they're partnered with store coupons you can really save a lot of money, and in many cases get items almost free. But, this tip comes with a warning. I have seen so many posts on social media of couponers bragging about their purchases and all I ever see is 20 packs of gum, 10 cases of spinach, 50 boxes of pencils and other exorbitant amounts of items that you may only need one or two of. Buying something simply because you have a coupon is not a good idea.

Never shop when you're hungry. Shopping when you are hungry is a sure way to give into temptation, compromise your food budget, and purchase items you don't need and are likely very unhealthy. Once you make it to the grocery store, I need you to shop as if your life depends on it, because it does. Go up and down each aisle and if you see something you'd like to purchase but is not on your list then put it on next week's list. Delay your gratification, it's okay you'll be fine; trust me. The only items you need to purchase that are not on your list or factored into your meal map are ingredient items that, if not purchased, would compromise the overall quality of the meal you're making.

**Start in the produce section.** Most large modern supermarkets have huge produce sections, often taking up a large portion of the store. Almost all fruits and vegetables are healthy, low in calories and delicious so here is where you can stock up. The most important thing to remember when shopping for fruits and vegetables is the old saw that variety is the spice of life; try a variety of different fruits and vegetables, including some you may never have heard of before to keep your meal plan fun and fresh. Some healthy-eating plans fail because they become boring and stale; but eating a variety of foods all but eliminates that hurdle.

**Buy your staples next.** Staple items are ingredients needed to complete your meals; seasonings, pasta, oils, salad toppings, gravies, sauces and the like.

**Read food labels…please!** Nutrition labels contain a wealth of information, but it is up to each shopper to read those labels and understand what they mean. Nutrition labels contain so much information; not just calories and fat content, but the amounts of various essential vitamins and minerals as well. It is important to know how to read labels in order to get the best nutritional bang for your food bucks.

**Pay close attention to packages sizes and brands.** Take advantage of the lower prices available on store brand and generic products. When it comes to packaging, watch out! Packaging can be deceptive, so get in the habit of comparing weights when shopping for canned fruits, vegetables and other items. For example, I recently purchased a bag of pre-packaged salad for $2.99, on sale for $2.99 per bag; the bag next to it was $2.50 on sale 2 for $5.00. I purchased the $2.99 bag of salad because the weight of the product inside had a value of $4.58 per pound while the other had a value of $8.00 per pound. I spent .49 cents more, but I got much more salad for the money I spent; even though the actual bags containing the salads were the same size. The colorful labeling hid the air occupying the top half of the sealed packaging of the more expensive bag of salad. Remember, manufacturers are banking on your tight schedule and lack of time to really comparison shop. They spend millions of dollars on focus groups and adjust their prices and packaging based on their findings.

**By the time you get to the meat section you should be half-way through your shopping list.** Buy the leanest cuts of meat you can find and if your store has a butcher ask if they can trim the fat from the edges of steaks, roasts and chops. Your goal should be 20-25 fat grams per day and if you're purchasing a fatty cut of meat you can easily hit your fat-gram limit in one item of one meal. Besides, the more fat on the meat, the more the piece of meat will cost. Even though poultry is generally low fat, not all poultry is created equal. Some varieties, like duck and goose, contain significant amounts of fat. A roast goose or duck can be great for Christmas or other special occasions, but these meats are generally too greasy to be eaten in everyday meals. Even low fat poultry like chicken breasts can benefit from some additional trimming. Removing the skin from chicken significantly cuts the amount of fat and calories it contains.

Additionally, using low fat white meat chicken instead of fattier dark meat is a smart move. My husband likes the skin on chicken so I actually buy regular chicken thighs with the skin and just peel it from my plate when I'm eating. Just because it's on my plate doesn't mean I have to eat it. When buying ground meats, always try to buy the leanest varieties you can afford. Ground beef that is 97% lean is a good choice. In addition, ground turkey or ground chicken makes a good, lower fat substitute for ground beef, and it can be used in all recipes that call for ground beef, including tacos, burritos, barbeque recipes and burgers. One important note about ground turkey and ground chicken, however; processed ground poultry products can contain surprisingly high levels of fat because manufacturers often grind up unwanted skin and fat in addition to the lean turkey or chicken. This is a particular problem with lower priced varieties of ground chicken and turkey, so it pays to read the labels and monitor the fat content carefully.

**Purchase baked goods, bread, dairy, cereals and snacks last.** Most grocery stores put snack items towards the front of the store and dairy items in the far back corner, this is strategic on their part. They want you to stock your basket with items they need to sell before you stock your basket with items that you actually need. Don't fall into their trap. Once your cart is filled with fruits, veggies, staples and meat then purchase your whole grains, snacks and dairy. Psychologically, at this point in your trip you should be fatigued; a few kids probably ran under your feet, chatty seniors got in your way in the seasonings aisle and your cell phone hasn't stopped ringing. By now you likely just want to be done and head home. That's why *now* is the perfect time to buy baked goods, bread, snacks and dairy, because you're too tired to pick and sort; you'll only buy what you need because you're ready to head home and hope the check-out line isn't 6 people deep. Buy whole grain breads and baked goods, they contain high amounts of fiber and other nutrients that more processed and refined baked goods lack.

When shopping for cereals in the grocery store, it is helpful to understand how the cereal aisle of the typical grocery store is arranged. Shelf space at a grocery store is in high demand and short supply, and cereal manufacturers take advantage of this fact in their store shelf marketing. In general, the less healthy, sugar-laden cereals are arranged at kid height, while the more adult, healthier products are on the top shelves. This is why your kids are always trying to put those sugar cubes disguised as cereal in your cart as you shop. Choosing the healthier cereals from the top shelves is a good strategy, but it is still important to read the labels to make sure you are getting what you think you are.

### Choose the healthiest frozen meals available

When it comes to eating healthy, freshly cooked food is always better, yet, in some cases it's impossible to cook a fresh meal every night. For people on the go, frozen meals can be healthy alternatives to fresh products. While there is no substitute for a well-balanced, home cooked meal using plenty of fresh and nutritious ingredients, healthy frozen meals can provide a quick and easy alternative for those who do not have time to cook meals from scratch. No matter what type of diet you're following, chances are there is a frozen meal available to meet your needs. From low fat to heart healthy to vegetarian meals, supermarkets offer great and varied options.

While frozen foods can be somewhat healthy, it's important to keep a close eye out for potentially, and sometimes buried, unhealthy ingredients. In particular, many frozen and prepared foods have unacceptably high levels of sodium and may use preservatives to which some people may be sensitive. Read food labels very carefully; these government-mandated labels contain a wealth of information and it's important to understand how the ingredients affect your personal fitness goals. I, along with dieticians, recommend keeping your daily sodium intake to less than 2300 milligrams per day; so when choosing a frozen meal make sure that one meal doesn't consume more than one-third of your daily suggested sodium intake. Making the claim "healthy" obligates food manufacturers to follow certain guidelines but its still up to smart consumers to review the labels and choose the healthiest options.

# Chapter Nine
# Time To Lose Weight!

You don't have to get it right, you just have to get it going
**Saideh Browne, Fitness Enthusiast and Media Entrepreneur**


This journey is all about you. What you put into it is exactly what you'll get out of it. I've spent most of my adult life as a media entrepreneur and as such, if I didn't work I didn't get paid. I respect people who have a job and sometimes I wish I were one of them. I don't get sick days, I don't get vacation days and I certainly don't get paid time off; if I'm not actively engaging in income and revenue generating activities I won't have money to pay my bills. This fitness experience was an exact replication of my career. If I didn't put in the work I didn't see the results. If you don't exercise and eat right you will not lose the weight – it's just that simple. You can't hire someone to do pushups for you. This is about you; and something you must do for yourself. **You don't get what you wish for, you get what you work for.**

There are no shortcuts on this journey. Hell, I wish there was a short-cut because I would have taken it. Laughingly, I must share with you how many times I've tried to cut 10 push-ups down to 8 during a personal training session – and you know what my trainer would do? He'd wait patiently until I hit 10 push-ups and only then would he let me proceed to the next circuit. Even if he would have let me stop at 8 push-ups I'd be the loser, not him. I wanted to lose weight so badly I bought books, hired a trainer, hired a weight loss coach and have maintained a gym membership for a few years now; I wanted a better life and this is the road I chose to get from where I was to where I wanted to be. I gave up happy hour with the girls, popcorn at the movies and home-baked chocolate chip cookies with my husband every night (yes, every night). I wanted my goal weight more than I wanted cookies, more than I wanted anything else in the world; it became a gentle obsession, and I am a better person for it. I am happier, I have more joy and I have more love to give because I have love for myself.

### ⭐ Weight loss is simple, but not easy

Weight loss, at its core is about eating less and moving more. We need to eat less, certainly, but it's just as important as moving more. I want you to be super-successful on your fitness journey; it's about being honest with yourself – your mind, body and soul. Getting fit requires mental strength and endurance; you'll never lose the weight if your mind is secretly betting against itself.

### ⭐ Losing weight is a marathon not a sprint

How many times have you started a diet only to fail a short time after? Many diets fail because we start them with false expectations. Crash diets, pills and other quick-fast solutions don't work. Well, actually they do but not for long. These programs don't focus on sustainable solutions and miss the opportunity to teach you how to eat, how to cook, how to shop for and prepare healthy meals; the whole training process is absent so when you become weak, there is nothing for you to fall back on. You don't have a base. Any major change in your life needs a solid foundation and those quickie plans are all fluff and air. There is nothing solid or sustainable about them. I can't stress enough how difficult this journey has been for me but because I took the long road and learned the basics I can and have committed to a healthy lifestyle. As of this writing, as evidenced by the photo of me on the cover of this book, I have not hit my goal weight but I'm damn sure working towards it and I won't be deterred. The holiday's and family gatherings make staying on track a little difficult but I have the support of family and my gym friends to keep me going.

When I laid out my plan and got the ball rolling to become more fit I had a pretty good idea of what my weight loss goal should be, based on my height, current weight and the weight I was when I was the most healthy in life. What I didn't do, and some do is, try to get back to the weight I was in high school. In high school I was 125 pounds which is far, far too thin for my 5'8" frame. I wasn't even a fully developed woman yet. We all need a little meat on our bones. As I began to lose weight I noticed that my body was slimming down but the scale wasn't moving enough – this is because I was losing fat and gaining muscle. You see 5lbs. of muscle and 5lbs. of fat both weigh 5lbs., the difference is that muscle takes up less space than fat so as I was losing fat the scale inched down; as I developed muscle the scale slowly inched back up thereby countering any weight loss. I was frustrated beyond measure, until I realized this was my body's response to my actions. It took time for me to fully grasp this concept but as I watched my body shrink it made a lot of sense.

After losing a good chunk of weight, I eventually plateaued and became frustrated again; the scale stopped moving even though my caloric intake decreased and my physical exertion increased. Out of sadness and feelings of failure, I gave up and went back to my old ways of eating. It took about a week and a half for the food I was eating to catch up to me. The first few days of my relapse the scale didn't move; even after about a week it had only gone up about 2 pounds. After about a week and a half I jumped on the scale and I was 6 pounds heavier! I thought, "What the hell?" and got right back on my grind. That's when I truly realized in order for this to work I could never go back to my old ways; and the only option was a complete life-long lifestyle change. I had to make permanent changes that I could live with day in and day out. Do I drink alcohol in the summer when I'm chilling on the beach? Yes, I do; but in moderation. Do I eat bowls of chili in the winter watching the football games with friends? Yes, I do; but in moderation and without excess cheese and sour cream and only if it's cooked with ground turkey and not ground beef or pork.. It's about taking small, incremental baby steps each and every time.

For some people, a healthy diet can be as simple as increasing the amount of fruits and vegetables they eat every day. For others, a radical change, involving strict control of fat and cholesterol, may be required. Even though every person will have different goals when it comes to healthy eating, the basic tenets are the same; with the most important being to eat a good variety of healthy foods, and eating less of the bad stuff. Chew your food slowly to help with weight loss. It takes your brain twenty minutes from the time you begin eating to send signals of being full. If you eat quickly, you often eat beyond your true level of fullness. Slow down, enjoy your meal, and you will be on your way to weight loss success.

This is a wild journey, and as women we must also include crazy hormonal swings, a monthly cycle and our tummy pooch that we may have to lift to shave down there. Hopefully after reading this book you won't have to lift anymore ☺. This book was written to help kick-start your fitness journey and I've shared some of the ups and downs of my journey with you. As we near the end of the book I want to highlight some of the tips that really got me over the humps when I needed help the most.

⭐ Don't use the scale as your only measure of success

A few days into my journey I jumped on the scale and was elated to see almost five pounds gone! That set a bad precedence; I thought if I did more of what I was doing then I'd keep losing weight so quickly. I was wrong; that initial weight loss was water and extra sludge in my system, I hadn't started losing fat yet. About a month into my journey none of my clothes fit, yet I was only down a few more pounds. My plan was working even though my results weren't reflecting on the scale. Don't use the scale as your only measure of success– use all of your faculties to gauge your progress!

⭐ Hygiene is very important

As you begin to exercise more your body will begin to absorb and release differently. You'll likely perspire more during the day and have the urge to drink more water. These changes coupled with the natural changes all women go through will require closer attention to hygiene. You may notice a different odor, you may sweat more between your legs and you may sweat more in other areas as well. If this is the case, take precautions to avoid embarrassing situations. Consider wearing panti-liners, use alcohol instead of deodorant or antiperspirant (it's cheaper, works better and won't stain your white shirts) and wear loose fitting clothes. Remember, this is not forever, it's just until you can get adjusted to the changes that are taking place as you become healthier.

⭐ Give your body time to adjust

Chances are it took many years to get to the weight you're at now; give your body time to get back to wholeness. When I joined my fitness program I was given a one year and a two year option. The one year option was a little more costly and intense so I opted for the two year option, even though as I was signing the contract I thought I was being hustled into two years of inescapable payments. I was wrong! I needed every bit of those two years. Half-way through year one I had emergency surgery on my appendix, because my program included a professional weight loss coach on speed dial I was able to maintain my nutritional program even though I couldn't make it to the gym. There are no short cuts to getting fit – it's about 100% dedication, 100% of the time. Don't be hard on yourself and give your body time to adjust to your new mindset and habits.

# Chapter Ten
# Enjoy The Journey!

Everything you see I owe to spaghetti.
**Sophia Loren, Academy Award winning Italian Actress**

Sophia Loren is widely known as one of the most curvaceous and sultry actresses ever and she is also known as an amazing cook as evidenced by the massive success of her published cookbooks. Sophia is Italian and her quote above, about owing everything to spaghetti, is so apropos for where you are in this book. You've read about calories, good foods, bad foods, how to grocery shop and even why yoga and meditation are so important, but through it all you must enjoy the journey…and a little pasta.

Here is the opening to a story I recently heard, and I'm sharing the gist of it with you.

*I was at work one day, calling on a customer who wasn't answering her phone. Her voice mail message started out in the usual way, "…we're not home, leave a message…" what followed was not so usual. It continued, "…by the way, we've recently made some changes in our life, if we don't call you back, you're one of the changes, beeeep".*

This approach is a little terse and I could never leave that as an outgoing message on my voice mail but I sure as hell would like to. The point is, whether you like her approach or not her message was clear. She changed her life

117

and didn't care who liked it or not. Change is never easy because it requires adjustments in areas that have given us comfort for so long. This woman was brave and you should be too.

Now that you have the knowledge and understanding that success on this journey is not overnight, you'll have a much better weight loss experience. Be patient and determined and you will succeed!

# Saideh's Final Thought

You don't get what you wish for, you get what you work for!

Love and Blessings,
Saideh

www.ingramcontent.com/pod-product-compliance
Lightning Source LLC
Chambersburg PA
CBHW031213270326
41931CB00006B/556